Read what fans of THE 40-30-30 FORMULA are saying:

"The most wonderful results occur on a daily basis: We find that we have greater mental clarity and more sustained energy throughout our days. The physical benefits are phenomenal."
                    —JERRY and LESLIE COOK, Post Falls, ID

"[The] recipes are wonderful! Just following the formula has made the weight literally drop off! I feel better than I have in years."
                    —BARB LAUB, Bloomington, IL

"My cholesterol went from a staggering 305 to 179. My body fat went from 22 percent to 16 percent. I have found a true way to control my weight and keep it down without sacrificing the foods I enjoy."
                    —NICOLAS TCHIKOVANI, Mountain View, CA

"I lost seventy-five pounds in twelve months. I used to wear a size twenty-two and now wear a size ten! I look ten years younger and feel ten years younger! Thanks to Gene and Joyce, I have a new lease on life."
                    —RENEE MCFERRON, St. Charles, MO

BY GENE AND JOYCE DAOUST

40-30-30 Fat Burning Nutrition

The Formula

Formula 101

FORMULA 101

MAINTAINING 40-30-30 NUTRITION FOR A LIFETIME

GENE AND JOYCE DAOUST

BALLANTINE BOOKS   NEW YORK

A Ballantine Book
Published by The Ballantine Publishing Group

Copyright © 2002 by Gene Daoust and Joyce Daoust

All rights reserved under International and Pan-American Copyright Conventions. Published in the United States by The Ballantine Publishing Group, a division of Random House, Inc., New York, and simultaneously in Canada by Random House of Canada Limited, Toronto.

Ballantine and colophon are registered trademarks of Random House, Inc.

www.ballantinebooks.com

Library of Congress Control Number: 2002095635

ISBN 0-345-45523-1

Manufactured in the United States of America

First Hardcover Edition: January 2002
First Trade Paperback Edition: January 2003

10 9 8 7 6 5 4 3 2 1

This book is dedicated to Joyce's brother, Rick Ruhmann,

a Florissant, Missouri, firefighter, and to all of this nation's brave firefighters.

Your daily concern for the lives of others often goes unnoticed.

But on September 11, 2001, we were all reminded of how often we forget to say thank you.

You all are true American heroes. Thank you.

CONTENTS

PART II: THE FORMULA 101 NUTRITION JOURNAL

APPENDIXES

ACKNOWLEDGMENTS

◇

We are truly fortunate that we have been able to work with an amazingly talented group of individuals. We would like to thank all of the doctors, pharmacists, trainers, nutritionists, athletes, and other health professionals that we acknowledged in *The Formula*. Without all of your support, the 40-30-30 nutrition revolution would not have happened.

We would also like to give special thanks to Randy Gage, Grant Teeple, Roland Frasier, Todd Hall, and the staff at Gage, Frasier and Teeple. Thank you for all of your work, guidance, and support.

Thanks to our agents, David Vigliano and especially Dean Williamson. And, of course, we give a special thanks to our editor, Maureen O'Neal, as well as Allison Dickens and Michelle Aielli at Ballantine Books. Your continued confidence in us has helped us to continue to develop 40-30-30 Formula nutrition programs that can help improve the lives of millions of people!

INTRODUCTION

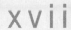

Gene and Joyce Daoust are nutritionists and authors of *40-30-30 Fat Burning Nutrition* and the national bestseller, *The Formula*. In the early 1990s, the Daousts worked closely with Dr. Barry Sears in developing and testing the original 40-30-30 zone nutrition program.

In 1992, the Daousts opened the BioSyn Human Performance Center, the world's first 40-30-30 zone nutrition clinic, located in Kirkland, Washington. They performed some of the original 40-30-30 nutrition studies at their clinic. It was there that they discovered how to make 40-30-30 nutrition easy to understand. They have a unique ability to inspire and motivate people from all walks of life to change their eating habits, lose weight, and improve their health. The Daousts were also the key nutritionists who helped to develop the nutrition programs for the leading 40-30-30 Nutrition Bar manufacturers.

The Daousts are dynamic speakers and motivational nutrition trainers and have become known as two of the nation's best nutrition coaches. Through the years, they discovered that people relied on them for encouragement, direction, and fresh ideas. *Formula 101* is designed to provide just that. *Formula 101* provides valuable, fresh, and easy-to-use information to help keep you motivated, confident, and focused. It contains many new recipes and is designed to teach you the necessary skills to easily maintain and follow the Formula 40-30-30 nutrition program for a lifetime. Whether your goal is to lose unwanted body fat, tone and shape up, or improve concentration and overall health, you'll enjoy and benefit from *Formula 101*.

UNDERSTANDING THE FORMULA

The Formula is the world's most complete and balanced nutrition program. It is a simple yet powerful nutrition plan designed for your specific requirements. Each meal and snack contains the 40-30-30 ratio of carbohydrate, protein, and fat designed to fuel your body correctly. The carbohydrate, protein, and fat ratio of a meal affects the balance of blood sugar, which regulates the hormonal effects of that meal.

High-carbohydrate diets elevate blood sugar and stimulate the release of the hormone insulin. Excess insulin forces the body to burn glucose rather than stored body fat for energy. Insulin stores glucose in the liver and muscles and converts excess glucose into fat.

High-protein diets can be even worse. Low-carbohydrate, high-protein diets deplete glucose and glycogen stores, resulting in ketosis. Ketosis is an abnormal metabolic process that breaks down protein and fat in an attempt to supply glucose to your brain. The body is forced to sacrifice body proteins and the incomplete fat metabolism creates ketone bodies that build up in the blood, upsetting the body's chemical balance. Headaches, dizziness, fatigue, nausea, muscle wasting, and continued low blood sugar are just a few of the possible unpleasant effects of a ketogenic diet. Urination is increased in an attempt to get rid of ketone bodies, leaching electrolytes and potassium. Initial weight loss can be primarily water weight at the expense of constipation, leg cramps, and muscle fatigue, not to mention the nasty smell of ketone gasses.

A balanced meal of carbohydrate, protein, and fat can help stabilize blood sugar levels, control insulin, and elevate the fat-burning hormone glucagon. Glucagon mobilizes stored glycogen in the liver to maintain and balance blood sugar levels and release stored body fat to be used as fuel.

The Formula is a balanced nutrition program that makes sense. The meals provide moderate amounts of carbohydrates (40%) to supply adequate glucose for your brain and to prevent ketosis. They provide adequate amounts of protein (30%) to supply amino acids needed to build and repair body proteins. Dietary protein releases the hormone glucagon, controlling insulin and maintaining blood glucose concentrations within a normal range for longer periods of time. Balanced meals also provide 30% "good fat." Fat is necessary to slow digestion and to further regulate blood sugar stabilization. It supplies the fatty acids required for appetite suppression and hormone production.

By eating the right proportion of carbohydrates, protein, and fat at each meal, you can begin to help your body automatically unleash its own natural fat-burning hormone, glucagon, while keeping blood sugar steady and energy levels high. The Formula has been personalized for your specific needs and body type. It is a dietary formula that your entire family can use for a lifetime.

THE FORMULA 101

1

KNOW YOUR PROTEIN REQUIREMENTS

◆

Protein is one of the six essential nutrients, along with carbohydrate, fat, vitamins, minerals, and water. Protein is classified as a macronutrient and must be consumed throughout the day. Protein foods are primarily those that come from an animal source. They supply the body with calories (4 per gram), as well as break down into amino acids. Amino acids build thousands of critical body proteins, including those necessary for hair, skin, nails, blood, hormones, digestive and regulatory enzymes, muscle tissue, brain neurotransmitters, and your immune system. Protein in every meal provides a continuous supply of amino acids and stimulates the release of glucagon, a fat-burning hormone that maintains stable blood glucose levels and releases stored fat so it can be burned for energy.

The Formula's revolutionary 40-30-30 nutrition ratio provides you with personalized nutrition plans that contain 30% of total calories from protein. Your sex, size, and activity level determine the amount of protein you need to maximize the burning of stored fat for energy. We have developed five different plans for you to choose from. When choosing the correct plan for your requirements, use your current actual weight, not your goal weight. For example, if you are a woman weighing 195 pounds and moderately active, choose the C plan. When your weight drops to 180 pounds, switch to the B plan.

Review the Formula Meal Plan Selection Chart to help you select the appropriate personalized meal plan and to determine your protein requirements. Now you know exactly how much protein you need for each meal and day. We know most people don't want to calculate the numbers at every meal, so we have done it for you in this book and in *The Formula*, with hundreds of meals and recipes designed for your personal protein requirements. So pick your favorite meals from the A, B, C, D, or E plan and you can be sure you are getting adequate protein for your individual protein requirements.

THE FORMULA
MEAL PLAN SELECTION CHART

W O M E N

Activity Level	Low–Moderate	Medium–High
Hours of Exercise per Week	Exercise 0–4 hours per week	Exercise 5–10 hours per week
Current Body Weight	*Use Meal Planner*	*Use Meal Planner*
Under 140	A	B
141–180	B	C
181–200+	C	D

M E N

Activity Level	Low–Moderate	Medium–High
Hours of Exercise per Week	Exercise 0–4 hours per week	Exercise 5–10 hours per week
Current Body Weight	*Use Meal Planner*	*Use Meal Planner*
Under 140	B	C
141–180	C	D
181–250+	C	D

Your Personalized Meal Plan is _____

THE FORMULA

MEAL PLAN SELECTION CHART FOR ELITE ATHLETES

FEMALE ELITE ATHLETES

Current Body Weight	Train 10 or more hours per week
Under 140	C
141–180	D
180 +	E

MALE ELITE ATHLETES

Current Body Weight	Train 10 or more hours per week
Under 140	C
141–180	D
180 +	E

Your Personalized Meal Plan is _____

THE FORMULA
PERSONALIZED PROTEIN REQUIREMENT CHART

Listed below are the total grams of protein for each meal plan tailored to individual requirements based on sex, weight, and activity levels.

Personal Meal Plan	A	B	C	D	E
BREAKFAST Protein grams	15	15	25	35	40
LUNCH Protein grams	20	30	30	40	50
SNACK Protein grams	15	15	15	15	30
DINNER Protein grams	30	35	40	40	50
DAILY TOTALS Protein grams	80	95	110	130	170

Your Total Protein Requirements:

BREAKFAST   LUNCH   SNACK   DINNER

_____   _____   _____   _____

2

STRETCH AFTER
EXERCISE

We used to think it was important to stretch *before* you exercise. Stretching before you run, play tennis, lift weights, or perform any exercise warms up your muscles. But new research is suggesting that stretching before exercise can decrease muscle strength and increase the risk of injury. One study showed that stretching decreased muscle strength for about 15 minutes. This study revealed that muscle electrical activity was decreased and the ability to turn on nerve-muscle fiber groups decreased with stretching. Several other studies in recent years also have shown that stretching prior to exercise decreases muscle strength.

But stretching is important. It promotes flexibility, reduces soreness, and relaxes the muscles you just used. Stretching also increases the range of motion in your joints and stretching after your workout reduces the risk of muscle strains, tears, and ruptures. Stretching is particularly important for strengthening tendons as you age. Yoga is a wonderful way to incorporate stretching along with meditation and mental concentration.

We recommend you devote approximately 30% of your total exercise time to stretching. So remember to stretch. It's best to stretch after exercise, when your muscles are warm and less vulnerable to injury.

3

SHARE YOUR RESULTS
WITH OTHERS

◆

When you begin to follow the Formula, it's a good idea to choose someone who cares about you and your health and share your success with him or her. Friends, relatives, or a spouse can be a great source of support. You may even want to report in weekly. The praise and encouragement you receive can be a wonderful source of motivation to keep you focused on your weight-loss goals. When you know you are looking and feeling great, the only thing better is to hear it from someone else.

When we had our clinic, many of our clients relied on us for praise and encouragement. But their weekly visits for weigh-ins and body fat testing were equally rewarding for us. As their body fat percentage dropped, they would tell us story after story of how their clothes felt baggy, their shoes no longer fit, their friends barely recognized them, and everyone wanted to know what they were doing. One woman, who used to refuse to tell anyone when she went on a diet, began to tell all of her friends that she gave up dieting for the Formula. Her enthusiasm and commitment to following the Formula was reinforced by sharing her results with others. Brad, Joyce's hairdresser, was so impressed with his results that he bought six books and gave them to friends.

Matt, one of our clients from the BioSyn Human Performance Center, used to tell everyone about his success. He lost more than 30 pounds of fat and gained 10 pounds of lean muscle in his first six weeks. He would enthusiastically explain how his previous high-carbohydrate bagel breakfast was the main reason he had gained weight and how his new, delicious 40-30-30 Formula Bagel Sandwich, which included cream cheese and turkey, was the reason he was finally burning fat and losing weight.

Try this delicious 40-30-30 Formula breakfast recipe. If it works for you as it has for us, Matt, and thousands of our clients, spread the word and share your results with others.

Breakfast

KIDS' FAVORITE

Bagel Sandwich

	MEAL PLAN PERSONAL REQUIREMENTS*				
	A	B	C	D	E
Bagel, plain, wheat, or oat bran, 3½-inch diameter	½	½	¾	1	1¼
Cream cheese, Philadelphia Brand lowfat	2½ tbsp.	2½ tbsp.	3½ tbsp.	5 tbsp.	6 tbsp.
or					
Cream cheese, full-fat	1¼ tbsp.	1¼ tbsp.	1¾ tbsp.	2½ tbsp.	3 tbsp.
Lean deli meat (turkey, chicken, or roast beef)	2 oz.	2 oz.	3 oz.	4½ oz.	5 oz.

DIRECTIONS: Spread toasted or untoasted bagel halves with cream cheese and top with sliced deli meat. *Note:* Choose amount from either lowfat or full-fat cream cheese.

For more than 200 personalized meals and recipes, including the Formula 40-30-30 Fat Flush Meals, refer to our book *The Formula*.

*To know your A, B, C, D, or E Meal Plan Personal Requirements, refer to Appendix A: The Formula Meal Plan Selection Chart.

4

STOP DIETING

Low-calorie diets, high-carbohydrate diets, juice diets, high-protein diets, the soup diets, the no-sugar diet. Forget them all. There have been hundreds of diets that promise weight loss, but most of them fail. Most diets are not balanced and can provide only temporary weight loss with possible undesirable side effects. Many are restrictive, difficult to follow, impossible to employ for a lifetime, and certainly not suitable for your entire family.

- **Low-calorie diets** deprive the user of essential nutrients and can result in constant hunger, blood sugar and hormonal imbalances, muscle wasting, and dry skin and hair.
- **The high-carbohydrate diets** can result in high or low blood sugar, hormonal imbalances, and muscle wasting. Inadequate protein intake can slow your metabolism so your body burns fewer calories and less fat. High-carbohydrate diets can leave you feeling hungry all the time and lacking energy. Long-term high-carbohydrate dieting can cause an increase in your fat-to-muscle ratio. You might weigh less, but you have gained fat and lost muscle.

- **Juice diets** are typically the same as high-carbohydrate diets and supply little or no protein and fat. They can cause blood sugar levels to surge, stimulating the release of the hormone insulin to lower them. Excess insulin prevents you from burning fat efficiently. Juice diets are far too restrictive and can be dangerous to follow for any length of time.

- **Food-combining diets** restrict you from eating many carbohydrates with protein. By eliminating protein at certain meals, they can result in hormonal imbalances and slow your metabolism. They are promoted to improve digestion, but poor digestion is usually due to a lack of digestive enzymes, not eating certain foods together. A balanced diet of 40% carbohydrate, 30% protein, and 30% fat at each meal helps supply all of the proper nutrients you need to build your digestive enzymes and improve your overall digestion.

- **The soup diets** have been popular for years but fail to supply adequate nutrients for a healthy body. These extreme, very-low-calorie diets can be inadequate in essential fats and protein. If your diet is too low in good fats and protein, it can trigger constant hunger, blood sugar imbalances, muscle loss, and dehydration. Extreme low-calorie diets are far too restrictive and impossible to follow for a lifetime.

- **High-protein diets** restrict carbohydrate intake. Low-carbohydrate diets can cause low blood sugar, hormonal imbalances, and ketosis. Ketosis can lead to muscle loss, body odor, and bad breath (from the ketone gases that ooze out of your body). High-protein diets also can be too high in fat, particularly the artery-clogging, saturated "bad" fat. They can cause sugar cravings, restrict many nutritious, high-fiber foods, and are difficult for you and your family to follow for any length of time.

So, stop dieting! Simply remove the word *diet* from your vocabulary and avoid following any nutrition plan that is not balanced. A healthy eating plan should:

- Recommend balanced amounts of carbohydrate, protein, and good fat.
- Provide personalized amounts for your specific size, sex, and level of activity.
- Be easy to use and suitable for your entire family to follow for a lifetime.

The 40-30-30 Formula is the nutrition solution to the dieting problem:

- The Formula *is balanced*, with 40% of total calories from carbohydrates, 30% from protein, and 30% from fat.
- The Formula *is personalized* for your individual requirements. Choose from the A, B, C, D, or E plan.
- The Formula *is easy* to use and provides precise meal plans that your entire family can use for a lifetime.

5

MEALS SHOULD
CONTAIN 30% FAT

The Formula promotes meals containing a balance of nutrients consisting of 40% of total calories from carbohydrate, 30% from protein, and 30% from fat. Your diet must supply adequate amounts of fat to obtain essential fatty acids. Essential fatty acids play a critical role in hormone balance, energy production, blood sugar stabilization, and hunger control.

When choosing foods that provide fat in a meal, look for fats that are unprocessed and occur naturally in foods, such as raw nuts and seeds, olives and avocados, and vegetable oils such as canola and olive oil. Fish also supplies a valuable source of fat that should be part of a healthy, balanced diet. It is wise to avoid fats known as *trans fats*. These are found in hydrogenated vegetable oils.

An important fact regarding fat is to remember that fat controls hunger. The fat in a meal actually slows the digestion of the meal so that it breaks down and enters the bloodstream more slowly, keeping blood sugar levels normal and signaling your brain that you are full.

A great example of the power of fat in a meal happened one day when Joyce was making the Berry-Peach Smoothie for lunch, only to discover that she was out of almonds. Because she already had it made, she drank it anyway, without adding an additional source of fat. Within the hour, her blood sugar was dropping and she was hungry. We were quickly reminded of the importance of fat in a balanced diet. She actually felt out of balance for the next several hours and vowed never to be without almonds again. In retrospect, she realized she could have eaten several olives or a slice of avocado. Don't forget the purpose of fat in your diet.

Lunch

KIDS' FAVORITE

Berry-Peach Smoothie

	MEAL PLAN PERSONAL REQUIREMENTS*				
	A	B	C	D	E
Strawberries, unsweetened, fresh or frozen	⅔ cup	1 cup	1 cup	1½ cups	1½ cups
Peaches, sliced, fresh or frozen	⅔ cup	1 cup	1 cup	1 cup	1½ cups
Water	½ cup	⅔ cup	⅔ cup	¾ cup	1 cup
Pure whey protein powder	15 grams	25 grams	25 grams	30 grams	45 grams
Granulated fructose	1 tsp.	2 tsp.	2 tsp.	2 tsp.	1 tbsp.
Almonds, sliced	1¾ tbsp.	2¾ tbsp.	2¾ tbsp.	3½ tbsp.	4½ tbsp.

DIRECTIONS: Combine all ingredients in a blender and process until smooth. *Note:* When making smoothies, we use pure whey protein powder. Whey protein powder is a natural protein from dairy. It is lactose and fat free, mixes instantly, and has a great amino acid profile. A high-quality whey protein powder should be 90% pure protein and contain no added sweeteners or flavors. For more information on pure whey protein powder, please refer to Appendix C: Special Ingredients. Granulated fructose is available at most health food stores and many grocery stores.

For more than 200 personalized meals and recipes, including the Formula 40-30-30 Fat Flush Meals, refer to our book *The Formula*.

*To know your A, B, C, D, or E Meal Plan Personal Requirements, refer to Appendix A: The Formula Meal Plan Selection Chart.

6

TRY 40-30-30 MEAL REPLACEMENT SHAKES

At least five studies published in the past two years confirm that substituting a low-calorie liquid meal for a regular meal is a good way to lose weight and keep it off. Scientists think that meal replacements are a good way to lose weight because they limit your choices, take the guesswork out of meals, and prevent overeating at that meal. Studies have also shown that thicker shakes are more satisfying. However, many of the meal replacement shakes available in stores are either high in protein, low in carbohydrates and fat, or high in carbohydrates and low in protein and fat. Their carbohydrate, protein, and fat content varies from flavor to flavor and they usually come in only one size. Continued use of shakes that are not balanced can cause muscle loss, dry skin, bad breath, constipation, hair loss, gallstones, and heart problems. Store-bought shakes contain preservatives, stabilizers, and unnecessary chemicals as thickeners and artificial flavorings.

We recommend making your own shakes and smoothies. 40-30-30 Formula shakes make following the plan easier and supply adequate protein, nutrients, fiber, and calories for the meal or snack being replaced. All of the Formula shakes contain the 40-30-30 ratio of carbohydrates, protein, and fat. We use a variety of carbohydrates, primarily from low-glycemic fruits. We believe pure whey protein powder provides the highest amino acid profile—far surpassing that of soy-based drinks. The fat is "good" fat from nuts and seeds, nut butters, or flax oil. And best of all, the Formula smoothies are delicious. Use frozen fruit or a little crushed ice for an even more satisfying, thicker texture.

The Formula contains personalized recipes for 22 smoothies and shakes, but we are always coming up with new flavors. Try some of these delicious new fruit smoothie recipes for breakfast.

Breakfast
Mango Magic

	MEAL PLAN PERSONAL REQUIREMENTS*				
	A	B	C	D	E
Mango, frozen	⅔ cup	⅔ cup	1 cup	1½ cups	1⅔ cups
Water, cold	⅔ cup	⅔ cup	1 cup	1¼ cups	1½ cups
Pure whey protein powder	15 grams	15 grams	25 grams	35 grams	40 grams
Granulated fructose	1 tsp.	1 tsp.	1½ tsp.	1½ tsp.	2½ tsp.
Macadamia nuts, chopped	1 tbsp.	1 tbsp.	1¾ tbsp.	2 tbsp.	3 tbsp.

DIRECTIONS: Combine all ingredients in a blender and process until smooth. Granulated fructose can be found in health food stores. *Note:* For more information on pure whey protein powder, please refer to Appendix C: Special Ingredients.

Breakfast
Mac Melon Smoothie

	MEAL PLAN PERSONAL REQUIREMENTS*				
	A	B	C	D	E
Honeydew melon, frozen	1 cup	1 cup	1¾ cups	2½ cups	3 cups
Water	⅔ cup	⅔ cup	1¼ cups	1½ cups	2 cups
Pure whey protein powder	15 grams	15 grams	25 grams	35 grams	40 grams
Granulated fructose	1 tsp.	1 tsp.	1½ tsp.	2 tsp.	2 tsp.
Macadamia nuts, chopped	1 tbsp.	1 tbsp.	1¾ tbsp.	2 tbsp.	3 tbsp.

DIRECTIONS: Use frozen melon balls or fesh melon, cubed and frozen. Combine all ingredients in a blender and process until smooth. *Note:* For more information on pure whey protein powder, please refer to Appendix C: Special Ingredients.

Breakfast
Macaloupe

	MEAL PLAN PERSONAL REQUIREMENTS*				
	A	B	C	D	E
Cantaloupe, cubed and frozen	1 cup	1 cup	1¾ cups	2½ cups	2¾ cups
Milk, nonfat	⅓ cup	⅓ cup	½ cup	⅔ cup	⅔ cup
Water	⅓ cup	⅓ cup	½ cup	⅔ cup	⅔ cup
Pure whey protein powder	15 grams	15 grams	20 grams	30 grams	35 grams
Granulated fructose	1 tsp.	1 tsp.	1 tsp.	1 tsp.	1½ tsp.
Macadamia nuts, chopped	1 tbsp.	1 tbsp.	1¾ tbsp.	2 tbsp.	3 tbsp.

DIRECTIONS: Use frozen melon balls or fresh melon, cubed and frozen. Combine all ingredients and process until smooth. *Note:* For more information on pure whey protein powder, please refer to Appendix C: Special Ingredients.

For more than 200 personalized meals and recipes, including the Formula 40-30-30 Fat Flush Meals, refer to our book *The Formula*.

*To know your A, B, C, D, or E Meal Plan Personal Requirements, refer to Appendix A: The Formula Meal Plan Selection Chart.

7

INCLUDE BEEF AS PART OF YOUR BALANCED DIET

Beef has been making a comeback after years of bad press regarding its cholesterol and saturated fat content. It's true that *lean* cuts of beef are a quality source of protein. Beef provides a complete source of amino acids and is particularly high in the muscle-building branch chain amino acids (BCAAs). Beef also is highly nutritious, supplying potassium, phosphorous, manganese, iron, creatine, and B Vitamins.

Choose lean cuts of beef and trim off any visible fat. Buy sirloin, trim well, and grind it for extra-lean sirloin burgers or use it in lasagna, sloppy joes, taco salads, and other recipes. You can even go one step further and buy drug-free, organically raised beef at health-conscious grocery stores or health food stores.

We've worked with many athletes through the years who intentionally avoided beef and ate primarily chicken, tuna, and vegetable protein sources. But when they complained of injuries, connective tissue damage, poor muscle strength, and flat muscle tissue, we immediately encouraged them to reintroduce red meats into their diet at least three to four times per week. The addition of adequate amounts of high-quality protein quickly provided the nutrients their bodies were lacking.

If you are a hard-training athlete or are having trouble building lean muscle mass, include lean cuts of red meat in your diet several times per week. Try this Kids' Favorite/Family Style dinner recipe for your active children. Sports and high activity levels leave their bodies starved for nutrient-dense, muscle-building meals.

Dinner

KIDS' FAVORITE/ *Family Style*

Sloppy Joes in Pita Pocket

	A	B	C	D	E
Sloppy Joes mixture (recipe below)	1 cup	1½ cups	2 cups	2 cups	2½ cups
Pita bread, wheat or white, 6½-inch size	1	1½	2	2	2½
Peaches, fresh sliced, or canned in water, drained	¾ cup	¾ cup	1 cup	1 cup	1½ cups

SLOPPY JOES RECIPE

2 tablespoons olive oil

½ cup minced onion

½ cup chopped celery

½ cup chopped green pepper

1 garlic clove, minced

1 pound ground turkey breast or extra-lean ground sirloin

½ cup chopped mushrooms

¼ cup bottled chili sauce

½ cup catsup

1 teaspoon Worcestershire sauce

½ cup water

RECIPE DIRECTIONS: Heat oil in skillet and sauté onion, celery, green pepper, and garlic until soft and just beginning to brown. Add ground meat and brown. Add mushrooms, chili sauce, catsup, Worcestershire sauce, and water. Simmer for 15 to 20 minutes uncovered.

DIRECTIONS: Spoon Sloppy Joes into pita bread halves and serve with peaches on the side.

For more than 200 personalized meals and recipes, including the Formula 40-30-30 Fat Flush Meals, refer to our book *The Formula*.

*To know your A, B, C, D, or E Meal Plan Personal Requirements, refer to Appendix A: The Formula Meal Plan Selection Chart.

8

ENTERTAINING WITH
THE FORMULA

We love to entertain, and part of being a responsible host or hostess is providing your guests with healthy foods from which to choose. Our guests always know there will be plenty of delicious, low-fat protein foods and balanced desserts when attending a party at the Daousts' house. High-protein appetizers can be eaten with high-carbohydrate alcoholic or nonalcoholic beverages. We also provide each guest with printed copies of several recipes that were served.

The following high-protein appetizers were the highlights of our 2000 Christmas cocktail party. Make these for your next elegant party. Healthy, 40-30-30 Formula food also makes for interesting conversation.

APPETIZER RECIPES

Sesame Chicken Skewers

4 large chicken breasts
Honey and pineapple teriyaki glaze marinade, bottled
¾ cup toasted sesame seeds

RECIPIE DIRECTIONS: Trim chicken of all fat. Cut each breast into ¼-inch thick slices. Trim the slices into 5-inch lengths x 1-inch wide strips. Thread one strip of chicken onto 6-inch skewers, piercing about 6 times to stretch along the length of the skewer, leaving about 1½-inch handle. Brush both sides with teriyaki glaze, cover and let marinate for 1 hour. Just before cooking, sprinkle both sides lightly with toasted sesame seeds. Place on a cookie sheet in even rows. Cover the exposed end of wooden skewers with a strip of foil to prevent burning. Place under broiler for 2 to 3 minutes on each side or until just browned.

DIRECTIONS: Serve hot or cold with bottled sweet and sour dipping sauce or soy sauce.

Smoked Salmon Egg Cups

12 eggs, hard-boiled
6 ounces smoked salmon
6 ounces Kraft Philadelphia Light Cream Cheese
1 diced green onion
1 teaspoon fresh lemon juice
Fresh dill, snipped

DIRECTIONS: Hard-boil one dozen eggs. Let cool, peel, and slice lengthwise. Discard yolks. Flake 4 ounces of salmon. Reserve 2 ounces of larger flakes for topping egg cups. Mix flaked salmon, cream cheese, green onion, and lemon juice. Spoon salmon filling into egg white cups, mounding slightly. Top with additional large flakes of salmon and sprinkle with snipped fresh dill. Any remaining salmon filling can be placed in the hollows of 3-inch long pieces of celery.

Crab-Stuffed Cherry Tomatoes

36 cherry tomatoes
12 ounces lump crab meat
3 tablespoons mayonnaise, reduced-fat
1½ teaspoons fresh lemon juice
¼ cup red bell pepper, diced
Salt and pepper to taste
Fresh basil leaves

DIRECTIONS: Wash and dry tomatoes. Slice ⅛ inch off the top of each tomato using a serrated knife. Scoop out the seeds with a small melon baller or grapefruit spoon. Mix crab, mayonnaise, lemon juice, red bell pepper, and salt and pepper to taste. Spoon crab mixture into tomato cups. Top with a small piece of fresh basil. Note: Cover a serving tray with an inch of shredded red leaf lettuce. This acts as a nest to hold the tomatoes in place.

Sliced Pork Tenderloin with Gourmet Mustards

Two 12-ounce roasted pork tenderloins with mustard glaze (recipe below)
Gourmet mustards:
    Spicy brown mustard
    Sweet honey Dijon mustard
    Horseradish mustard
    Jalapeño mustard

MUSTARD GLAZE
½ cup prepared mustard
¼ cup maple syrup
1 teaspoon salt
½ teaspoon ground black pepper

DIRECTIONS: Preheat oven to 450°F. Mix together prepared mustard, maple syrup, salt, and pepper. Rub the glaze over entire surface of the pork tenderloins and cook to an internal temperature of 150°F to 155°F. Remove from the pan to cool and refrigerate. Slice pork into ¼-inch slices and serve with several different prepared gourmet mustards.

For more than 200 personalized meals and recipes, including the Formula 40-30-30 Fat Flush Meals, refer to our book *The Formula*.

9

TRY WHEY
PROTEIN POWDER

In all of our smoothie recipes and many of our desserts, we include whey protein powder as part or all of the required 30% protein. After years of research and trial and error, we highly recommend the use of this superfood. Once chalky and barely tolerable, protein powders have evolved to this newest generation. Although there are many types of protein powders (soy, egg and milk combinations, egg white, vegetable, and milk), we feel that pure whey protein has many advantages. Pure 90% whey protein contains a superior amino acid profile and virtually zero carbohydrates or fat, mixes easily, can be used in baking, and has a pleasant taste. It is derived from dairy but is lactose-free and contains no added sweeteners or flavors.

When shopping for a pure whey protein powder, use Gene's 90% rule: Look at the label to determine the serving size (in grams) and multiply by .90. The number you get should be the same as the total grams of protein listed in the nutritional information on the label. There should be less than one (<1) gram or zero grams of carbohydrate or fat per serving. Look for a pure whey protein powder with the following nutritional profile:

PURE WHEY PROTEIN POWDER

Nutritional Profile

Serving size	1 scoop (22.2 gram size)
Calories	80
Carbohydrate	0 grams
Protein	20 grams
Fat	0 grams

Whey protein is not just for making smoothies. Although we have many smoothie recipes in this book and in *The Formula*, you can also add whey protein powder to almost anything that can be mixed, blended, or stirred. Try this thick and creamy Chocolate Peanut Butter Shake dessert recipe. It is so delicious you would never know it is a healthy, balanced 40-30-30 Formula recipe.

DESSERT RECIPE

KIDS' FAVORITE

Chocolate Peanut Butter Shake

¾ cup lowfat vanilla frozen yogurt

⅓ cup nonfat milk

2 teaspoons natural peanut butter

1 tablespoon unsweetened cocoa powder

15 grams pure whey protein powder

DIRECTIONS: Combine frozen yogurt, milk, and peanut butter in a blender and process until smooth. Add cocoa powder and whey protein powder and blend. Pour into two small glasses and serve at once. Makes two servings. *Note:* For more information on pure whey protein powder, please refer to Appendix C: Special Ingredients.

Per serving: 170 calories; Grams = C-17.5g, P-13g, F-5.25g

For more than 200 personalized meals and recipes, including the Formula 40-30-30 Fat Flush Meals, refer to our book *The Formula*.

10

HAVE ONLY ONE STARCHY FOOD PER MEAL

Through the years, we have seen that the number-one problem most people have with losing weight or burning fat as efficiently as possible is that they eat far too many starchy carbohydrates. One of the simplest things you can do to help your body burn more stored fat is to have only one starchy food per meal. You don't have to give up these delicious foods, simply cut back on the bread, rice, potato, or pasta at each meal. Instead of having several different starches, choose only one starch per meal.

Starchy foods like chips, crackers, pretzels, breads, rice, pasta, and potatoes are very dense sources of carbohydrates. They pack an incredible amount of carbohydrates per serving. For example, 1/2 cup of rice, pasta, or potatoes has more than 20 grams of carbohydrates, compared to 1/2 cup of broccoli with about 5 grams of carbohydrates. Even worse, starchy foods are very high-glycemic foods. High-glycemic foods increase blood sugar quickly (which is not good, if your goal is to lose weight and burn fat). If blood sugar rises too much or too fast, the hormone insulin is released to lower it. Excess insulin prevents the burning of stored body fat. Even worse, excess insulin can convert a majority of the excess glucose into fat and store it in your fat cells. So, if you are eating a lot of starchy foods, even though they are fat-free, many of those carbohydrates will be converted into fat and stored away.

Here's a great way to reduce the starches when eating out in a Mexican restaurant. Order either chicken or fish fajitas *without* the rice or beans. Pass on the chips and have the fajitas and grilled vegetables with one or two tortillas. Because you also need a little fat, you can even have a small amount of guacamole or sour cream.

Starchy foods are less expensive than protein, so many restaurants serve large portions of starchy carbohydrates for economic reasons. Mexican restaurants can be the most challenging because of all of the starchy carbohydrates that are typically served. But instead of having chips, rice, beans, and tortillas, simply choose one of these and turn a potentially weight-gaining, fat-storing meal into a fat-burning meal.

You can see how these simple adjustments allow you to still enjoy many of your favorite foods. Use the one-starch method when eating out at any restaurant or when preparing your own meals. You don't have to deprive yourself—it is simply a matter of balance.

11

DON'T BE AFRAID
OF GOOD FAT

For years, you have heard that dietary fat makes you fat: If you reduce your dietary fat consumption, you will not gain weight or get fat. An overwhelming belief in that concept gave birth to an entire new food industry of fat-free cookies and snacks, ice cream, and yogurt. But after 20 years of following this advice, Americans have gotten fatter. Many of the manufactured fat-free foods were loaded with carbohydrates. It was such a powerful marketing concept that many foods that never even had fat in them were marketed as fat-free.

But, you might ask, how can beer make you fat? It doesn't contain fat, yet we've all heard of beer bellies. A 12-ounce beer has approximately 150 calories, less than one gram of protein, 13 grams of carbohydrates, and zero grams of fat. The remaining 98 calories are from alcohol. When alcohol is consumed, it is converted into glucose (carbohydrates), so beer is virtually 100% carbohydrates. If you drink six beers, that's an extra 900 calories of pure carbohydrate. These calories are the kind that rapidly enter your bloodstream and cause blood sugar levels to spike. High blood sugar inhibits your fat cells from releasing fat, and excess calories and glucose get converted into and stored as fat. So, even though beer is fat free, the excess carbohydrates found in beer and many other high-carbohydrate foods are getting you fat. The same problem occurs with sugary sodas and drinks. They don't contain fat, but are loaded with high-glycemic, blood-sugar-spiking, insulin-raising, fat-storing carbohydrates. In our opinion, sugary drinks are one of the main causes for the shocking rise in obesity and diabetes in this country, especially in children.

Good fat not only tastes good (sliced avocado tastes great in a sandwich), but it's good for you. Forget everything you've heard about fat being bad for you. Good fat is good for you. Listed below are a few facts about fat.

Good fats:
- Control carbohydrate metabolism. Fat in a meal controls blood sugar levels.
- Provide satiety. Fat in a meal eliminates hunger from meal to meal.
- Provide essential fatty acids, "the building blocks of eicosanoids" (your master hormone regulators).

Eat several different kinds of fat in moderation. Did you know that it is healthier to sauté your vegetables in a little butter than in most vegetable oils or margarine (saturated fats found in butter withstand high heat better than other fats). You can have up to 10% of your total calories from mono-unsaturated fats, 10% from polyunsaturated fats, and 10% from saturated fats. This balance is not only good for you, but makes following a healthy eating plan easy to follow as well as delicious.

Some of the best good fat sources include:

- Raw nuts and seeds
- Olives and avocados
- Coldwater fish, such as salmon and tuna
- Olive oil

Just remember: Good fat doesn't make you fat.

12

HAVE YOUR OWN PERSONAL AFFIRMATIONS

Affirmations are phrases you say to yourself that help you proclaim your goals and desires. They serve as instant reminders to stay on track. We have found personal affirmations to be very helpful when following the Formula. They define your mission and assist you in developing new eating habits and healthy food choices. They keep you focused and are even helpful during exercise. Think of your affirmation as a simple reminder for your brain to tell your body what to do. Thinking positive thoughts paints vivid images and helps your subconscious motivate you to reach your deepest desires.

An affirmation can either be a statement, such as *I'm a strong, powerful person*, or just a few words, such as *calm, relaxed, in control*. Begin by choosing powerful words that are personal to you and will help you achieve your goals. For instance, if you binge eat, choose *control*; if you are stressed, choose *calm*; if you are in poor health, choose *strong* or *healthy*. Once you come up with a personal affirmation that suits you, repeat it often during the day. Write it down and put a copy on the refrigerator, in your bedroom, and on the bathroom mirror. Soon it will just pop into your head and become your instant reminder to keep your diet balanced.

Gene has several personal affirmations: *calm*, *relaxed*, *in control*, and *lean*, *mean*, *fat-burning machine*. During his workout, he replaces counting repetitions with repetitive words. Because words have meaning, he is tapping into the mind-muscle connection and is able to stay much more focused during his workout.

Joyce's affirmations include *healthy*, *balanced*, and *body fuel* while she prepares meals. She repeats *strong*, *lean*, and *gorgeous legs* while she runs or walks. It really helps keep her focused on her goals and can work as easily for you.

Here are several suggestions to get you started in developing your own personal affirmations:

- *Stable, strong, calm, control*
- *Control, balanced, burning fat*
- *I'm a strong, powerful person.*
- *I control food, it doesn't control me.*
- *Delicious, balanced, in control*
- *Strong, toned, fit*
- *Focused, positive, feeling great*
- *Size, shape, hard, ripped* (good for a bodybuilder)
- *Toned, lean, beautiful curves* (good for a woman)
- *Smooth, strong, buns of steel*

Talk to yourself. When it's positive, it's motivational.

Write in your personal affirmations here:

" _____ "

" _____ "

13

LEARN THE POWER OF MAKING HEALTHY EATING CHOICES

Every time you eat a meal or snack, you have the choice to eat a healthy, balanced meal or not. Whatever your choice, you will live with the hormonal consequences of that meal for the next four to six hours. With a better understanding of the physical consequences of food, you can begin to make better food choices every time you eat.

- Did you ever notice that after eating donuts for breakfast, you feel sleepy at work?
- Have you ever felt lethargic after a big pasta lunch?
- Do you seem to munch on everything you can get your hands on before dinner?

These are typical reactions to low blood sugar caused by eating high-carbohydrate meals. But if you learn to control blood sugar from meal to meal, you can begin to eliminate those sleepy mornings, lethargic, foggy afternoons, and out-of-control evening bingeing.

When you eat a balanced ratio of carbohydrate, protein, and fat at each meal, you help your body automatically unleash its own natural fat-burning hormone, glucagon, the key to getting rid of unwanted body fat while keeping blood sugar steady and energy high. You can actually control the way your body burns fat through the hormonal response you create with every balanced meal or snack you eat.

A diet high in carbohydrates can elevate the fat-storing hormone insulin. Elevated insulin levels are also directly linked to diseases such as hypertension, hyperlipidemia, type II diabetes, and obesity. The Formula's revolutionary caloric ratio of 40% carbohydrates, 30% protein, and 30% fat gives you the power to help control your insulin levels with the foods you eat. Balanced nutrition becomes your direct link to longevity and helps provide the nutrition solution to living a healthy life and feeling the best you can feel.

Mark, one of our clients, remarked that because he exercised, he thought could eat anything he wanted. But he was always feeling tired and was short-tempered with his employees. He also measured 20% body fat and had trouble building muscle. He was glad to finally understand that his food choices were the real cause of his problems. In only one week of following the 40-30-30 Formula, he experienced dramatic changes. He began to use a wonderful affirmation: "Food no longer controls me, I do." His energy level improved as well as his mood.

When Mark understood how powerful his food choices were in controlling his ability to burn fat, lose weight, and build muscle, it was easy for him to give up junk food and start making healthy eating choices.

If you're not happy with how you feel or perform, don't give up. Simply start making healthy food choices at every meal. Balanced meals will help you control the hormonal effects of food.

14

TAP INTO YOUR GROWTH HORMONE

Mention human growth hormone (HGH) and everyone thinks of athletes who want to increase muscle size and strength. But HGH is not only the most anabolic hormone in your body for building muscle, it promotes the growth and repair of all body tissues, including the formation of antibodies. It is an important metabolic hormone that helps make fat available for fuel. New studies are showing that HGH appears to improve the strength of the heart muscle in heart failure patients as well as lower blood fats that contribute to hardening of the arteries.

Growth hormone:

- Keeps muscles strong and toned.
- Strengthens the heart.
- Burns body fat for energy.
- Slows the aging process.

As children, we have plenty of HGH to help us grow and build strong, healthy bodies, but as we age, our production of this hormone begins to decline. However, research on athletes has shown that intense exercise increases the release of HGH. As muscle tissue is torn down, additional growth hormone is required to repair it. Have you ever noticed that people who work out on a regular basis seem to look younger? HGH is also an anti-aging hormone. When you add up all the benefits of HGH, it makes sense to include some intense exercise in your workout routine.

You can tap into your own natural source of HGH through exercise and a balanced diet. A diet high in carbohydrates elevates insulin levels and blocks the release of HGH. If you have been carbohydrate-loading before your workout and drinking high-carbohydrate drinks during your workouts, you may be unknowingly blocking HGH release and minimizing the benefits you should be getting from exercise.

Denise, one of our clients, complained of slow muscle recovery and poor muscle tone. She did aerobics daily and lifted weights three times per week but said it was impossible for her to tone her muscles. Her skin appeared wrinkled and saggy and very dull. Her muscle tone was almost nonexistent. Upon analyzing her diet, we discovered she was a "carbohydrate junkie." She avoided fat and ate very little protein. In fact, after reviewing her diet more closely, the only protein she was consuming was primarily from vegetables and very little fish or chicken a few times a month. An amino acid analysis showed her deficient in many amino acids, but particularly leucine, isoleucine, and valine (the three branch chain amino acids responsible for muscle growth), and lysine and proline, important in tendon and connective tissue.

We immediately changed her diet to include adequate amounts of high-quality protein from eggs, chicken, lean beef, fish, and whey protein powder. She began eating 30% of her total calories in good fats such as olive oil, raw nuts and seeds, and avocados. Denise had followed the For-mula for seven days when she returned to report unbelievable improve-ments. She claimed that her muscles felt like they were full after being empty for years, her energy was tremendous, and her mood swings disap-peared. She couldn't believe the improvement in the texture of her skin. She said she felt seven years younger in only seven days and finally realized the power of a balanced diet. After following the Formula for more than a year, she looks at least ten years younger and loves her new lifestyle. By tap-ping into HGH and balancing her diet along with exercise, Denise believes she has found the formula for the fountain of youth.

So, tap into your own natural source of HGH with exercise and a bal-anced diet.

15

USE AN
EXERCISE BALL

Exercise of any kind burns calories, increases your metabolism, tones and builds muscles, and improves cardiovascular health and circulation. Exercise makes you healthier and more fit, and makes you feel better. But the most powerful effects could be the hormonal benefits of exercise. When you exercise, you lower insulin (the fat-storing hormone), increase glucagon (the fat-burning hormone), and release human growth hormone (the building and repairing hormone). Exercise, along with following a balanced diet like the 40-30-30 Formula, can finally produce the kind of fat-burning results you hoped for.

New research is showing that you should combine aerobic and anaerobic exercise with stretching for a well-rounded workout to achieve the best fitness and weight-loss results. We developed a 40-30-30 workout system that we have been using for years. It is a method to help you easily incorporate all three forms of exercise into the time you can devote to your workout. Here's how it works: Spend 40% of the total time you can work out on aerobic exercise, 30% on anaerobic exercise, and 30% on stretching. For example, if you exercise for 40 minues per day, spend 16 minutes doing aerobic exercises like running or walking, 12 minutes doing anaerobic exercises like push-ups, sit-ups and squats, and 12 minutes stretching . You will find the time flies by and your workouts never get boring. And the good news is that you don't have to do it all at once—you can break it up throughout the day. Try 16 minutes walking in the morning, 12 minutes doing push-ups and sit-ups in the evening, and 12 minutes stretching before bed.

We recommend a variety of exercise and have recently begun using an exercise ball. These are large rubber balls filled with air that come in various sizes. The exercise ball is great for stretching, or it can provide an intense workout with a greater range of motion. The best thing about the ball is that you can do both stretching and resistance training with one exercise. Even just sitting and balancing on the ball requires the stabilizer muscles in your back to contract and helps tone the abdominal muscles. Try sitting on the ball for an hour while you are working on your computer or watching televison. A new survey of more than 500 ACE-certified private trainers voted crunches on an exercise ball as the best ab exercise. We keep our 29-inch ball in our family room and use it often for stretching out and strengthening the back, many different ab exercises, and basic sitting to improve posture and balance.

THE 40-30-30 EXCERCISE FORMULA
Gene and Joyce's
40-Minute Excercise Ball Workout

40% Aerobic   16 minutes power walk or run.

30% Anaerobic   Choose 3 to 4 strength exercises and do 3 to 4 sets of 8 to 12 repetitions for each exercise.

30% Stretching   Choose 3 to 4 stretching exercises using the exercise ball.

Note: Review the directions that are supplied with your ball for proper execution of each exercise. Do not start this or any exercise or nutrition plan before consulting with your doctor or health care practitioner.

For variety and an awesome workout, try getting on the ball. You and your entire family will enjoy using it.

16

INCLUDE EGGS IN YOUR DIET

◆

For years, eggs were given a bad rap because they contain choles-terol, and nutrition and health experts urged us to eliminate them from our diet. But new research confirms what we've been saying for years: that elevated insulin levels from high-carbohydrate diets can ele-vate cholesterol far more than having a few eggs as part of a balanced diet.

So, welcome back the egg. Eggs are an excellent source of protein. In fact, eggs are the highest-quality protein found in nature. Eggs are not only high-quality protein, but they are a rich source of essential fats, Vitamins A, D, and E, thiamine, riboflavin, pantothenic acid, folic acid, Vitamin B-12, biotin, phosphorus, manganese, iron, iodine, copper, calcium, and zinc. The whole egg is also an excellent source of the essential amino acids, spe-cifically, the sulfur-bearing amino acids that are powerful antioxidants and help fight free-radical damage.

The egg white is pure protein, and the egg yolk contains both fat and protein (the protein in the yolk is primarily sulfur-bearing amino acids). A medium-size egg contains less than 1 gram of carbohydrate, 5 grams of pro-tein, and 4 grams of fat. The fat is 60% of the total calories of the egg, but that fat isn't all bad; 38% is monounsaturated and 14% is polyunsaturated.

And, to compensate for the fat and cholesterol, the yolk contains lutein and zeaxanthin, carotenoids that protect the eyes and protect against colon cancer. Discarding the yolk in an attempt to remove some of the fat removes about half of the protein and primarily the sulfur-bearing amino acids. The sulfur aminos are powerful detoxifiers. So, when using eggs in a meal or recipe, remove some of the yolks to lower the fat content, but keep one or two to maintain the amino acid profile of the egg and all of the nutrients and health benefits they supply. Besides, eggs taste a whole lot better and are much more appealing when they are a little yellow.

Eggs are one of the most economical sources of protein. One dozen eggs cost about $1.35 and provide a whopping 60 grams of high-quality protein. Compared to fish, chicken, or beef (all of which are lower-quality proteins), eggs are quite a bargain. Also, now available are the new super-eggs: The hens have been fed special feed and lay eggs with increased Omega-3 fatty acid content.

We like to hard-boil a dozen eggs each week so we always have a quick, fresh, and natural source of high-quality protein ready to peel and eat. Try the following breakfast recipe the next time you crave eggs, and forget all of the terrible things you've heard about eggs. Eggs as part of a balanced diet are not only good, they're good for you.

Breakfast

KIDS' FAVORITE

Scrambled Eggs and Toast

	MEAL PLAN PERSONAL REQUIREMENTS*				
	A	B	C	D	E
Eggs, whole	1	1	1	2	2
Egg whites only	2	2	4	5	6
Bread, reduced calorie, whole wheat, toasted	1 slice	1 slice	2 slices	2 slices	2 slices
Whipped butter	1 tsp.	1 tsp.	2 tsp.	2 tsp.	1 tbsp.
Preserves, any flavor	1 tsp.	1 tsp.	1 tsp.	2 tsp.	2 tsp.
Orange, medium size	½	½	½	1	1½

DIRECTIONS: Scramble eggs and whites in a nonstick pan. Spread toast with whipped butter and preserves. Serve eggs and toast with fresh orange sections.

For more than 200 personalized meals and recipes, including the Formula 40-30-30 Fat Flush Meals, refer to our book *The Formula*.

*To know your A, B, C, D, or E Meal Plan Personal Requirements, refer to Appendix A: The Formula Meal Plan Selection Chart.

17

LEARN PORTION CONTROL

The Formula is a nutrition program that is personalized for your individual requirements. There are five distinct meal plans—A, B, C, D, and E—that have been developed to fit your individual needs. By choosing the correct plan, you will learn portion control to enhance fat loss. Too much food will slow weight loss, but too little food will slow your metabolism and just as easily inhibit fat loss. Adequate calories are vital for weight loss and longevity.

Your sex, actual body weight, and level of activity determine the overall amount of food and the number of calories you need daily to maximize the burning of stored body fat.

A married couple came to our clinic back in 1992. The husband weighed 265 and did little exercise and his wife weighed 215 with moderate exercise. They were instructed to both follow the C plan. That meant they were both to eat identical meals. After two weeks, they returned to our clinic. He had lost 18 pounds and was feeling great. She had lost only 4 pounds, was hungry, moody, and ready to give up. She said that she followed the plan exactly for both of them. It was only when her husband revealed that she was following the A plan in a desperate attempt to lose weight faster that we discovered her problem. She was not eating enough for her size. We convinced her that more food was the solution. One week later, she called to say she felt much better. She no longer experienced hunger between meals, and her clothes were beginning to hang on her. When her weight reached 180 pounds, we reduced her calories slightly by switching her to the B plan while her husband remained on the C plan. They both continued to lose weight and were feeling great.

They reached their ideal weight and have learned the importance of portion control for their individual requirements. The Formula is now their way of eating for a lifetime.

THE FORMULA
MEAL PLAN SELECTION CHART

W O M E N

Activity Level	Low–Moderate	Medium–High
Hours of exercise per week	Exercise 0–4 hours per week	Exercise 5–10 hours per week
Current body weight	*Use Meal Planner*	*Use Meal Planner*
Under 140	A	B
141–180	B	C
181–200+	C	D

M E N

Activity Level	Low–Moderate	Medium–High
Hours of exercise per week	Exercise 0–4 hours per week	Exercise 5–10 hours per week
Current body weight	*Use Meal Planner*	*Use Meal Planner*
Under 140	B	C
141–180	C	D
181–250+	C	D

Your Personalized Meal Plan is _____

THE FORMULA
MEAL PLAN SELECTION CHART FOR ELITE ATHLETES

F E M A L E   E L I T E   A T H L E T E S

Current Body Weight | Train 10 or more hours per week

Under 140   C

141–180   D

180+   E

M A L E   E L I T E   A T H L E T E S

Current Body Weight | Train 10 or more hours per week

Under 140   C

141–180   D

180+   E

Your Personalized Meal Plan is _____

18

SATISFY THOSE
CRUNCHY CRAVINGS

Food cravings tend to come in two flavors—sweet or salty. Sweet cravings are easier to address when following the 40-30-30 ratio by eating fruit with cottage cheese and nuts or a variety of smoothie recipes found in this book or *The Formula*. *The Formula* also contains many dessert recipes as well as recommending the use of 40-30-30 Nutrition Bars and Shakes that you can buy in a variety of flavors and that satisfy any sweet craving.

More challenging are the salty or crunchy cravings. Foods like chips, popcorn, and pretzels are either predominantly carbohydrates or carbohydrates with fat. They are typically highly processed and high-glycemic and contain trans fatty acids. Following is the nutritional profile of many popular crunchy snack foods.

SAMPLE NUTRITIONAL PROFILE OF CRUNCHY SNACK FOODS

	Calories	Carbohydrates	Protein	Fat	Glycemic Rating
1 ounce of potato chips	150	15	2	10	High
1 ounce of pretzels (sticks)	110	23	2	0	Very high
¼ cup unpopped popcorn	180	36	6	2.5	Very high
3½ cups popped popcorn with butter	150	19	3	11	Very high
3 cups light popped popcorn	65	10	1.5	2.5	Very high
1 ounce white corn tortilla chips	140	19	2	6	High
2 rice cakes	70	14	2	0	Very high

If you choose to include crunchy snacks, do so in moderation. Many of our clients have helped us come up with some delicious 40-30-30 Formula crunchy snacks. Try these the next time you want a balanced snack to satisfy a crunch attack.

Snack

Chips and Dip

	MEAL PLAN PERSONAL REQUIREMENTS*				
	A	B	C	D	E
Cottage cheese, 2% lowfat	½ cup	½ cup	½ cup	½ cup	¾ cup
Salsa	3 tbsp.	3 tbsp.	3 tbsp.	3 tbsp.	5 tbsp.
Corn tortilla chips, white or yellow	¾ oz.	¾ oz.	¾ oz.	¾ oz.	1⅓ oz.

DIRECTIONS: Mix cottage cheese and salsa. Serve as a dip with chips.

Snack

Pretzels and Cheese Snack

	MEAL PLAN PERSONAL REQUIREMENTS*				
	A	B	C	D	E
Pretzel sticks	½ oz.	½ oz.	½ oz.	½ oz.	1 oz.
String cheese, lowfat	1 oz.	1 oz.	1 oz.	1 oz.	2 oz.

DIRECTIONS: Have pretzel sticks with cheese.

Snack

Chips and Tuna Snack

	MEAL PLAN PERSONAL REQUIREMENTS*				
	A	B	C	D	E
Potato chips, baked (Lays or Ruffles)	1 oz.	1 oz.	1 oz.	1 oz.	2 oz.
Tuna salad, deli-style	3 oz.	3 oz.	3 oz.	3 oz.	6 oz.

DIRECTIONS: Have chips with tuna salad.

For more than 200 personalized meals and recipes, including the Formula 40-30-30 Fat Flush Meals, refer to our book *The Formula*.

*To know your A, B, C, D, or E Meal Plan Personal Requirements, refer to Appendix A: The Formula Meal Plan Selection Chart.

19

DON'T SKIP YOUR MIDAFTERNOON SNACK

The Formula recommends eating four meals per day: breakfast (within one hour of waking), lunch, (approximately 4 to 5 hours after breakfast), a midafternoon snack, and dinner. It is generally a good idea to eat every 4 to 5 hours to maintain stable blood sugar levels throughout the day. Some diet experts recommend that people eat many small meals during the day instead of three large ones. But new research is showing that the danger of eating many small meals throughout the day is that people end up eating too many calories during a 24-hour period.

If you are following the C plan, your daily protein requirements are 110 grams and 1,465 calories. If you skip the midafternoon snack, you will be missing 15 grams of protein or approximately 200 calories for that day. If you ate lunch at 12 noon and dinner at 7:30, you have gone for 7 1/2 hours without refueling your body and reprogramming your fat-burning hormones. Your blood sugar and energy levels will surely dip and can lead to overeating at dinner. If you do this only occasionally, don't worry. But if you do this on a regular basis, you may notice hunger and cravings return and a slowdown in your rate of fat loss, either from consuming too few or too many calories.

So, instead of skipping that midafternoon snack and slowing down your body's natural fat-burning process, take the time to have a balanced snack. It's a great way to take a break from a hectic day, and by eating a Formula snack, you will be reprogramming your hormones to burn fat efficiently.

Enjoy these delicious snacks that are easy to prepare.

FORMULA 40-30-30 FAT FLUSH
MEAL PLAN PERSONAL REQUIREMENTS*

Snack

KIDS' FAVORITE
String Cheese and Grapes

	A	B	C	D	E
String cheese, lowfat	2 oz.	2 oz.	2 oz.	2 oz.	4 oz.
Grapes, green or purple	¾ cup	¾ cup	¾ cup	¾ cup	1½ cups

DIRECTIONS: Have cheese with grapes.

MEAL PLAN PERSONAL REQUIREMENTS*

Snack

Deli Tuna Salad on Apple Slices

	A	B	C	D	E
Tuna salad (prepared with lowfat mayonnaise)	3 oz.	3 oz.	3 oz.	3 oz.	6 oz.
Apple, medium	1	1	1	1	2

DIRECTIONS: Spoon deli-style tuna salad onto apple slices.

For more than 200 personalized meals and recipes, including the Formula 40-30-30 Fat Flush Meals, refer to our book *The Formula*.

*To know your A, B, C, D, or E Meal Plan Personal Requirements, refer to Appendix A: The Formula Meal Plan Selection Chart.

20

EAT MORE SALMON

This powerhouse of seafood is a quality source of protein. We eat salmon two to three times per week. One 4-ounce cooked portion of salmon provides about 30 grams of protein. It is easy to digest and contains high amounts of the essential amino acids, particularly the sulfur amino acids, powerful detoxifiers, and immune-building nutrients. Salmon also is high in the essential amino acid lysine.

That same 4-ounce portion of salmon supplies approximately 11 grams of fat, of which 55% is monounsaturated (the "good" fat). Salmon is one of nature's highest sources of the superfat EPA. EPA is an Omega-3 fatty acid that is very healthy to have in your diet but is sometimes hard to get. These fats help reduce heart disease and support the immune system.

Salmon is an excellent source of B Vitamins, which are essential for your body's production of energy, and help you cope with stress. Salmon is an exceptionally high source of Vitamin B-12, used in the metabolism of carbohydrates, protein, and fat and a known reducer of homocysteine blood levels, which also lowers the risk of heart disease. It supplies a good balance of phosphorous and calcium, needed to prevent bone deterioration.

This superfood, known as a functional food, provides so much more than calories. It is one of nature's most nutrient-dense, perfect foods. Its nutrients give you energy and help fight disease and aging. Try the following easy-to-prepare Grilled Salmon Dinner recipe. It is one of our favorites and is sure to become one of yours. Make salmon part of your balanced eating plan for a lifetime of good health.

Dinner

MEAL PLAN PERSONAL REQUIREMENTS*

Grilled Salmon Dinner

	A	B	C	D	E
Salmon steak or fillet	4 oz.	5 oz.	6 oz.	6 oz.	7 oz.
Red potatoes, 2½-inch diameter, cooked	1⅓ cup	1½ cup	2 cups	2 cups	2½ cups
Asparagus spears, steamed	10 spears	10 spears	10 spears	10 spears	12 spears
Mixed salad greens	2 cups	2 cups	2 cups	2 cups	2½ cups
Italian salad dressing, full-fat	2 tbsp.	2 tbsp.	2 tbsp.	2 tbsp.	2½ tbsp.

DIRECTIONS: Broil or grill salmon steak. Season with salt, pepper, garlic, and lemon juice to taste. Serve with cooked red potatoes, steamed asparagus, and a green salad with dressing.

For more than 200 personalized meals and recipes, including the Formula 40-30-30 Fat Flush Meals, refer to our book *The Formula*.

*To know your A, B, C, D, or E Meal Plan Personal Requirements, refer to Appendix A: The Formula Meal Plan Selection Chart.

21

THINK GUILT-FREE: IT'S OKAY

I t's time to remove the word *guilt* from your vocabulary. Most diets restrict foods to the point that if you stray, you've blown your diet and feel guilty. Because no one likes to feel he or she has done something wrong, it's easier to just give up. How many times have you binged, only to decide to start your diet over again on Monday?

The Formula is a personalized eating plan that takes the guesswork out of eating and removes the guilt. The revolutionary balance of 40% carbohydrates, 30% protein, and 30% fat eaten at every meal is intended to help stabilize blood sugar, help control insulin, and elevate your fat-burning hormone glucagon to improve your ability to burn fat efficiently from meal to meal. If you occasionally binge and eat too many carbohydrates, don't worry. You should actually feel relieved to know that as quickly as your next meal, you can correct the hormonal imbalance and get back on track. In fact, we encourage clients to occasionally binge on high-carbohydrate foods just to remind them how they can make you feel.

Lynn, one of our clients, works in an office with many employees. Each Friday afternoon, management orders an extra large sheet cake with all of the names of those celebrating birthdays for that week. When Lynn began following the Formula, she was determined to be "perfect," as she called it, so she celebrated with her coworkers but politely declined the cake. After losing 50 pounds and feeling better than ever, she decided it was time to indulge. One Saturday morning she phoned to tell us she ate birthday cake at work that Friday afternoon in place of her 40-30-30 snack. She described how guilty she felt while eating it and how quickly her blood sugar levels spiked, then crashed, leaving her lethargic, out of focus, and with a headache. She was surprised to experience such a powerful reaction to a food she once ate without these effects. We explained that by following the Formula for the past several months, her body adjusted to feeling balanced on a regular basis. Eating a large, sugary slice of cake is an easy way to remind yourself how good the Formula makes you feel. Lynn no longer feels guilty if she chooses to indulge. She knows the hormonal imbalance will last only a short while.

Go ahead and splurge once in a while. It's nothing to feel guilty about. Just return to the 40-30-30 Formula at your next meal and you'll be back on track, feeling great, and burning fat.

22

IF YOU EAT TOO MANY CARBOHYDRATES, EXERCISE

◆

When you follow the Formula you begin to learn proper portion control for your personal requirements. But what should you do if you eat too many high-glycemic carbohydrates in a meal? Simply adding additional protein and fat in an attempt to balance the meal will only increase the total calories of that meal. Eating a meal that is high in carbohydrates can elevate blood sugar, stimulating the release of insulin. Your body has no choice but to burn the glucose from the carbohydrates you just ate for energy, blocking the release of stored body fat. This will occur until the excess glucose is either burned or stored. You can correct the hormonal imbalance at your next meal, but you also have one other choice to help mop up the excess glucose and insulin: exercise.

Exercise lowers insulin levels while using the excess glucose for energy. Although fat is the preferred source of fuel for muscles, if blood sugar levels and insulin are high, your body's only source of fuel will be glucose. But don't get in the habit of relying on exercise to lower high blood sugar levels. Exercise is a powerful tool for burning unwanted body fat, but a balanced diet is even more so. If your diet is balanced and blood sugar is stable before you begin to exercise, you can burn stored body fat as your primary source of energy during your workout and experience the kind of results you expect.

Jeff is one of our clients who used to follow a high-carbohydrate, low-fat diet, and he exercised daily. He combined both cardiovascular and weight training, but no matter how much exercise he did, he couldn't get that hard, "ripped" look he wanted. His high-carbohydrate diet was simply sabotaging hours of exercise. When he began following the Formula, his blood sugar was balanced, thereby controlling insulin (the fat-storage hormone) and increasing glucagon (the fat-mobilization hormone). In as little as two days, Jeff noticed improved strength in his training sessions and a much fuller muscle pump (that's weight-training-speak for a fuller, thicker, stronger feeling in the muscles). Within two weeks, he was noticeably leaner, more vascular, and had much better muscle definition. He commented that he had no idea that getting a great body could be as easy as changing his diet. Jeff combines the Formula with exercise for the hard body he always wanted.

It's best to follow the Formula with regular exercise. But if you occasionally overeat on carbohydrates, additional exercise can help you burn the extra glucose and get you back on track.

23

MAKE A 40-30-30 FORMULA DESSERT

Most desserts are high in carbohydrates, fat, or both. But we have developed delicious desserts that contain 40% of calories from carbohydrate, 30% from protein, and 30% from fat. Making 40-30-30 desserts is easy, delicious, and can be part of your balanced dietary plan.

To convert a dessert recipe into a 40-30-30 dessert, review the carbohydrate, protein, and fat ratio of the original recipe. Desserts high in sugar and flour will be harder to balance without altering the taste and texture too much. Cookies and cakes are very challenging. But desserts that are protein-based, such as cheesecakes, puddings, custards, and ice cream, are easy to modify and still taste great. You will find many delicious dessert recipes in this book and in *The Formula*. The following are key points to remember when developing your own favorite recipes:

- If a recipe calls for eggs, reduce the fat and increase the protein by using two to three egg whites for each whole egg.
- Replace high-glycemic sugar with fructose, a granulated fruit sugar that is very low-glycemic. Fructose can be found in most health food stores in the bulk food bins or bags.

- You can generally reduce the fat in a recipe by one third to one half and use canola oil in place of saturated fat. However, we're still having trouble with cookie recipes.

- Use pure whey protein powder to increase the protein in a recipe.

One of our favorite dessert recipes is Rich Chocolate Pudding. It requires no cooking or baking and can be made in as little as 10 minutes.

KIDS' FAVORITE/ *Family Style*

Rich Chocolate Pudding

10½ ounces lowfat silken tofu

½ teaspoon vanilla

1½ tablespoons natural creamy peanut butter

2 tablespoons cocoa powder

2½ tablespoons granulated fructose

10 grams pure whey protein powder

DIRECTIONS: In a small food processor, blend tofu on high until creamy. Add vanilla and peanut butter and blend for 30 seconds. Add cocoa powder and fructose; mix gently with a spatula, then blend for 1 minute, opening the processor to scrape the sides. Mix in the protein powder and blend for 1 minute, scraping sides if needed. Measure equal portions into 4 small cup servings and cover with plastic wrap before refrigerating. Makes 4 servings. This recipe can be doubled if using a full-size food processor. Note: For more information on pure whey protein powder, please refer to the Appendix at the back of the book.

Per serving: 130 calories; Grams = C-12.5g, P- 9.75g, F-4.5g.

For more than 200 personalized meals and recipes, including the Formula 40-30-30 Fat Flush Meals, refer to our book *The Formula*.

24

INDULGE IN THE FORMULA CHEESECAKE DIET

If you love cheesecake, then you've found your dream diet. Regular cheesecake is high in carbohydrate and fat and could never be thought of as a diet food. But cheesecake with a 40-30-30 ratio not only is delicious, but can be enjoyed on a regular basis when following the Formula.

We developed the New York Style Cheesecake because thick, rich cheesecake has always been one of our favorite desserts. After weeks of trial and error, we finally came up with a recipe that was perfect: smooth and creamy and, best of all, rich and delicious. We served the cheesecake at dinner parties and shared the recipe with friends. One day, we saw a close friend who had lost 20 pounds. She informed us that she was following our "cheesecake diet." Two months earlier, she had attended one of our dinner parties, where we explained that the delicious cheesecake they were raving about was 40-30-30 Formula-approved. It was actually no different from eating a 40-30-30 Nutrition Bar or a balanced Formula meal. She decided that if there was no difference, she could simply replace a meal or snack for equal amounts of Formula cheesecake. She said her favorite meal replacement was breakfast and she felt great all morning after eating it. She ate Formula meals for lunch and dinner, but admitted that many days, she would have cheesecake again for her midafternoon snack. And so, the Formula Cheesecake Diet was born.

But it gets even better: The carbohydrates used in the cheesecake recipes are low- to medium-glycemic, making them Formula 40-30-30 Fat Flush approved.

THE FORMULA CHEESECAKE DIET

You can replace breakfast with the appropriate amount of cheesecake for your personal requirements. Have a 40-30-30 Formula meal for lunch and dinner. You have the option of a slice of cheesecake or a Formula snack midafternoon. If you stay up late, you may prefer to eat your midafternoon snack several hours after dinner.

SCHEDULE

Breakfast	Formula Cheesecake
Lunch	Formula meal
Snack	Formula Cheesecake or snack
Dinner	Formula meal

FORMULA 40-30-30 FAT FLUSH
MEAL PLAN PERSONAL REQUIREMENTS*

Breakfast

	A	B	C	D	E

KIDS' FAVORITE/ *Family Style*

New York Style Cheesecake

	A	B	C	D	E
New York Style Cheesecake (recipe below)	1⅓ slices	1⅓ slices	2⅓ slices	3 slices	3¾ slices

FORMULA 40-30-30 FAT FLUSH
MEAL PLAN PERSONAL REQUIREMENTS*

Snack

New York Style Cheesecake

	A	B	C	D	E
New York Style Cheesecake (recipe below)	1⅓ slices	1⅓ slices	1⅓ slices	1⅓ slices	2⅔ slices

NEW YORK STYLE CHEESECAKE RECIPE

16 ounces Philadelphia Brand Fat-Free Cream Cheese

16 ounces Philadelphia Light Whipped Cream Cheese

¾ cup granulated fructose

2 large eggs

1 egg white

2 teaspoons vanilla

1 cup fat-free sour cream

1 tablespoon cornstarch

50 grams pure whey protein powder

RECIPE DIRECTIONS: Preheat oven to 325°F. Lightly grease and flour a 9-inch springform pan. In a large mixing bowl, beat together cream cheese and fructose until light. Add the eggs and egg white, beating thoroughly after each. Blend in vanilla and sour cream. Add the cornstarch and whey protein powder and mix well. Pour the mixture into the pan. Place a pan with 1 inch of hot water on the bottom rack of the oven. Bake the cake at 325°F for 45 minutes on the center rack. It is recommended that you use a timer. Turn off the oven without opening the door and let cake cool for 1 hour. Let cake cool thoroughly before unmolding. It's normal for the cake to crack slightly.

To unmold, carefully run a knife between the cake and pan rim and release the sides of the springform pan. Serve plain or decorate with sliced strawberries, kiwi, or raspberries. Cake can be stored covered with plastic wrap in the refrigerator for up to 10 days, or frozen. Makes 16 servings. *Note:* For more information on pure whey protein, please refer to the Appendix at the back of the book.

Per slice: 150 calories; Grams = C-15g; P-11g; F-5g.

*To know your A, B, C, D, or E Meal Plan Personal Requirements, refer to Appendix A: The Formula Meal Plan Selection Chart.

25

HOW TO SPLURGE ON HIGH-CARBOHYDRATE DESSERTS

I f you are planning a night out to celebrate a birthday or anniversary, remember this advice on how to enjoy dessert while you keep your diet
balanced. The Formula promotes the 40-30-30 ratio at each meal to
stabilize blood sugar throughout the day. If you have been following the
personalized meals in *The Formula,* you should have a pretty good idea of
the proper balance of foods on your plate. A Regular Formula dinner contains the appropriate serving of protein, a large serving of vegetables, one
serving of starchy carbohydrates, and a salad with dressing. But if you
would like to have dessert without overeating, adjust your meal to avoid
eating the starchy carbohydrate food.

Order grilled or baked chicken breast with steamed vegetables and a
dinner salad with dressing. Drink water, iced tea, or a glass of sparkling
mineral water with a slice of lime. So far, your meal contains protein from
the chicken, a very small amount of carbohydrates from the vegetables and
lettuce, and a small amount of fat from the dressing. You actually haven't
eaten enough carbohydrates and you need dessert in order to balance your
40-30-30 ratio. The carbohydrates found in a potato, rice, or white bread
are no different from those found in a sugary dessert. They are equally

high-glycemic and all carbohydrates convert into glucose. But, because you ate primarily protein from the chicken first, it will act as a buffer to slow down the digestion of the dessert and help reduce the potential rise in blood sugar.

The following example is based on the personal requirements for dinner found in the C and D plans.

Approximate dinner requirements: 53 grams of carbohydrate, 40 grams of protein, and 18 grams of fat.

SAMPLE DINNER	CARBOHYDRATES	PROTEIN	FAT
5-ounce chicken breast	0	32	3
Steamed green vegetables (1 to 2 cups)	6	3	0
Dinner salad (mixed greens)	2	1	0
Italian salad dressing (1 tablespoon)	0	0	4
Mineral water with lime	0	0	0
Total	8	36	7
Add:			
Chocolate mousse cake	38	2	10
Nonfat latte with a cube of brown sugar	7	4	0
New Totals	53	42	17

You can choose from a variety of different desserts and add a nonfat latte.

DESSERT EXAMPLES	CARBOHYDRATES	PROTEIN	FAT
Tiramisu	39	3	13
Vanilla layer cake with icing	41	2	13
Devil's food layer cake with icing	40	2	14

DESSERT EXAMPLES	CARBOHYDRATES	PROTEIN	FAT
Chocolate mousse cake	38	2	10
Chocolate mousse	34	3	8
Cherry pie	43	3	14
Pumpkin pie	40	5	11

Remember, meals don't have to be exactly 40-30-30: close is good enough. So go ahead and splurge on special occasions. If you are going to indulge in high-carbohydrate, high-fat desserts, eat lowfat protein and minimal carbohydrates in your meal first.

26

BALANCING SUMMER PICNICS

Summer is certainly the time to be in great shape and have lots of energy. Yet, when we go to the beach, we notice that people are eating primarily junk food. It's easy to believe the latest statistics that 61% of Americans are overweight and that a full 26% are either obese or grossly overweight. Summertime events should be no excuse to overeat. In fact, it's even more important to eat healthy, balanced meals so you can be fit and enjoy all of the activities. Rather than coolers full of sugary sodas and beer and bags of chips and candy, you can plan 40-30-30 Formula meals and snacks that are delicious and satisfying and even suit the occasion. Follow these helpful tips when planning your outdoor meals.

Choose lowfat protein foods, such as:

- Grilled chicken skewers
- Deviled or hard-boiled eggs
- Sliced turkey or chicken breast
- Chicken strips in hot sauce
- Tuna salad
- Lowfat cheese cubes or string cheese

Choose from a variety of carbohydrate foods, such as:

- Fruits: grapes, berries, cherries, apples, peaches
- Crunchy vegetables: edible pea pods, celery sticks, red and green pepper strips, dill pickle spears. Bring a lowfat vegetable dip.
- Pretzel sticks or baked chips

Choose from a variety of quality fats, such as:

- Black or green olives—try a mixture of Greek olives.
- Mixed nuts in the shells (you eat fewer that way)—bring a nutcracker.

The following is a sample of the 40-30-30 Formula meal we served our guests on the Fourth of July.

FOURTH OF JULY MENU

Turkey sandwiches

Grapes

Edible pea pods

Red and green pepper strips

Dill pickles

Mixed Greek olives

Sparkling water

Lunch

	MEAL PLAN PERSONAL REQUIREMENTS*				
Whole Wheat Turkey Sandwiches	A	B	C	D	E
Whole Wheat Turkey Sandwich (recipe below)	1/2	3/4	3/4	1	1 1/4
Grapes, red or green seedless	8	10	10	20	20
Snap peas, edible pod	5	8	8	8	10
Red and/or green bell pepper strips	5	5	5	5	5
Dill pickle spear	1	1	1	1	2
Mixed Greek olives, large	1 1/2	2	2	2	3

Dinner

	MEAL PLAN PERSONAL REQUIREMENTS*				
Whole Wheat Turkey Sandwiches	A	B	C	D	E
Whole Wheat Turkey Sandwich (recipe below)	3/4	3/4	1	1	1 1/4
Grapes, red or green seedless	10	10	20	20	20
Snap peas, edible pod	6	8	8	8	10
Red and/or green bell pepper strips	5	5	5	5	5
Dill pickle spear	1	1	1	1	2
Mixed Greek olives, large	2	2	2	2	3

WHOLE WHEAT TURKEY SANDWICH RECIPE

1 whole wheat roll, 6 inches long

1½ tablespoons reduced-fat mayonnaise

1 tablespoon prepared mustard

1 tablespoon olive oil and vinegar salad dressing

1 thin slice sweet onion, white or red

3 thin slices of tomato

5 thin slices of cucumber, peeled

1 leaf of red leaf lettuce

2 diced pepperoncinis

4 ounces sliced deli-style turkey breast

1 ounce sliced deli-style Swiss cheese, lowfat

Salt and pepper to taste

RECIPE DIRECTIONS: Slice roll lengthwise and remove most of the soft inside bread, decreasing the carbohydrates by about one third and making room for the filling. Spread the hollowed-out inside of one half with reduced-fat mayonnaise and mustard and drizzle the other half with salad dressing. Place diced pepperoncinis, thin slices of onion, tomato, and cucumber and the lettuce on one half and turkey and cheese on the other. Sprinkle with salt and pepper. Combine both halves and wrap tightly with plastic wrap.

DIRECTIONS: Serve sandwich with grapes, edible pea pods, red and green bell pepper strips, dill pickle, and olives. Serve with sparkling water or any sugar-free beverage.

For more than 200 personalized meals and recipes, including the Formula 40-30-30 Fat Flush Meals, refer to our book *The Formula*.

*To know your A, B, C, D, or E Meal Plan Personal Requirements, refer to Appendix A: The Formula Meal Plan Selection Chart.

27

FOLLOW THE FORMULA 40-30-30 FAT FLUSH TO HELP YOU BURN FAT FASTER

◇

The Formula 40-30-30 Fat Flush is a personalized dietary plan developed to help you speed up weight loss and maximize fat burning. It was originally developed in our clinic for bodybuilders and competitive athletes to follow for six weeks prior to competition. Although rather restrictive, the athletes would lose body fat quickly without sacrificing lean muscle mass. The results were so outstanding, we developed a less restrictive plan for our clients to follow.

Each Formula Fat Flush meal contains the 40-30-30 ratio of carbohydrates, protein, and fat, but the carbohydrate sources are only low- to medium-glycemic foods. Carbohydrate foods are virtually all plant foods. They provide direct energy for your brain, central nervous system, and muscle cells in the form of glucose or blood sugar and are classified as simple or complex. Newer research includes the glycemic index of carbohydrate foods. This is a measure of how much and how quickly a food affects blood sugar. Simple sugars that enter the bloodstream very quickly and cause a large spike in blood sugar have a high-glycemic rating. Low-glycemic carbohydrate foods contain a higher percentage of fiber or protein and have a milder effect on blood sugar. Your body secretes the hormone insulin when faced with a rapid increase in blood sugar. Insulin promotes the storage of fat. When blood sugar is steady, the hormone glucagon is elevated to help you naturally burn stored body fat faster.

The Formula 40-30-30 Fat Flush can be used for several weeks at a time or for a lifetime. It includes a wide variety of healthy foods to choose from. The low- to medium-glycemic carbohydrates include fruits such as berries, peaches, plums, pears, citrus, and apples. When following this plan, avoid bananas and dried fruits, which are high-glycemic. Vegetables such as asparagus, cauliflower, broccoli, cabbage, tomatoes, onions, green beans, sweet potatoes, peppers, and salad greens are some of your best carbohydrate choices, along with grains like barley and bulgur. These low- to medium-glycemic fruits, vegetables, and grains provide significant sources of Vitamins A, C, and E, beta-carotene, folic acid and folate, selenium, bioflavonoids, and antioxidants. They are packed with fiber, phytochemicals, and cardioprotective nutrients. Avoid starchy vegetables and grains like corn, potatoes, white rice, pasta, and bread, which are high-glycemic.

Follow the Formula 40-30-30 Fat Flush plan for 21 days. There are 100 breakfasts, lunches, snacks, dinners, and desserts to choose from. Choose from the A, B, C, D, or E personalized plan suitable for your individual requirements. The following is a sample day of Formula 40-30-30 Fat Flush meals.

ONE-DAY SAMPLE OF THE FORMULA 40-30-30 FAT FLUSH MEALS

MEAL PLAN PERSONAL REQUIREMENTS*

Breakfast	A	B	C	D	E
Eggs and Bacon					
Eggs, whole	1	1	1	2	2
Eggs, whites only	1	1	1	2	2
Canadian bacon	1 oz.	1 oz.	2 oz.	2 oz.	3 oz.
Tomato, medium, sliced	½	½	1	1	1
Grapefruit sections with juice	⅔ cup	⅔ cup	1 cup	1⅔ cups	2 cups

DIRECTIONS: Scramble, hard-boil, or poach eggs. Serve with heated Canadian bacon, sliced tomatoes, and grapefruit sections.

MEAL PLAN PERSONAL REQUIREMENTS*

Lunch	A	B	C	D	E
KIDS' FAVORITE					
Tuna-Lettuce Wraps and Fruit					
Albacore tuna, water-packed and drained	4 oz.	6 oz.	6 oz.	8 oz.	10 oz.
Celery, diced	½ stalk	½ stalk	½ stalk	1 stalk	1 stalk
Green onion, diced	1	1	1	1	1
Red cabbage, finely shredded	⅓ cup	⅔ cup	⅔ cup	1 cup	1 cup
Italian bottled salad dressing, full-fat	1½ tbsp.	2½ tbsp.	2½ tbsp.	3 tbsp.	¼ cup
Lettuce leaves, romaine or red leaf	2	4	4	6	7
Apple	1	1	1	2	2½
	medium	large	large	medium	medium

DIRECTIONS: Combine tuna, celery, onion, cabbage, and Italian salad dressing. Divide tuna mixture and roll in lettuce leaves. Serve with apple slices.

Snack

Lowfat Cottage Cheese and Fruit

	MEAL PLAN PERSONAL REQUIREMENTS*				
	A	B	C	D	E
Knudsen On the Go! Lowfat Cottage Cheese and Fruit (4 oz. cup)	1	1	1	1	2
Nuts (almonds, pecans, or walnuts)	1 tsp.	1 tsp.	1 tsp.	1 tsp.	2 tsp.

DIRECTIONS: Mix cottage cheese and fruit with nuts.

Dinner

Beef Stir-Fry with Barley

	MEAL PLAN PERSONAL REQUIREMENTS*				
	A	B	C	D	E
Beef Stir-Fry (recipe below)	$1\frac{1}{2}$ cups	$1\frac{2}{3}$ cups	$1\frac{3}{4}$ cups	$1\frac{3}{4}$ cups	2 cups
Pearl barley, cooked	$\frac{2}{3}$ cup	$\frac{2}{3}$ cup	$\frac{7}{8}$ cup	$\frac{7}{8}$ cup	$1\frac{1}{8}$ cups

BEEF STIR-FRY RECIPE

$1\frac{1}{2}$ pounds beef tenderloin

3 tablespoons soy sauce

3 tablespoons dry cooking sherry

1 clove garlic, pressed

1 teaspoon ground ginger

1 teaspoon red pepper flakes

4 cups chopped broccoli

4 cups sliced asparagus (2-inch slices)

2 cups mushroom pieces

$1\frac{1}{2}$ tablespoons cornstarch

1 cup beef broth, canned

2 tablespoons peanut oil, divided

RECIPE DIRECTIONS: Trim beef of visible fat and cut into $\frac{1}{2}$-inch wide $\times$ 2-inch long strips. In a bowl, mix beef strips, soy sauce, sherry, garlic, ginger, and pepper flakes. Cover and refrigerate for at least 20 minutes. Heat 1 tablespoon of the peanut oil in a skillet or wok over high heat. Stir-fry beef mixture until browned; remove from pan. Add the remaining peanut oil to wok and stir-fry the broccoli and asparagus for about 3 minutes or until vegetables are tender-crisp. Add mushrooms for about 1 minute more. Blend cornstarch and beef broth in a small bowl and add to vegetables, stirring until sauce boils and thickens.

DIRECTIONS: Serve Beef Stir-Fry over hot cooked barley.

For more than 200 personalized meals and recipes, including the Formula 40-30-30 Fat Flush Meals, refer to our book *The Formula*.

*To know your A, B, C, D, or E Meal Plan Personal Requirements, refer to Appendix A: The Formula Meal Plan Selection Chart.

28

SCHEDULE YOUR MEALS
TO FIT YOUR LIFESTYLE

40-30-30 Formula meals should be eaten every four to five hours. Breakfast meals intentionally contain fewer calories than lunch and lunch contains fewer calories than dinner only because the majority of people we work with have become accustomed to eating that way. If you would rather eat a larger lunch and a smaller dinner, by all means, adjust meals to fit your lifestyle preferences.

To adjust the meal plans found in this book and in *The Formula*, begin by determining your personal requirements. For example, if you follow the C plan, your total daily requirements are:

Total daily requirements—C Plan
Carbohydrate—146 grams
Protein—110 grams
Fat—49 grams
Total daily calories—1,465

TOTAL MEAL REQUIREMENTS—C PLAN

	Breakfast	Lunch	Snack	Dinner
Carbohydrate grams	33	40	20	53
Protein grams	25	30	15	40
Fat grams	11	14	6	18
Total Calories	331	406	194	534

If you prefer to have a larger lunch than dinner, follow the D lunch and have the A portion for dinner. Because your lunch was larger, you may not require the midafternoon snack between lunch and dinner. You can have it earlier in the day or as an afterdinner snack. Several of our clients work very early hours or graveyard shifts. If you work unusual hours, consider the first meal you eat after waking as breakfast. Be certain to eat every four to five hours to maintain stable blood sugar levels throughout the day.

Michael, one of our clients and a computer programmer, began work at 4:00 A.M. He worked long hours, and often didn't leave work until 4:00 P.M. Before he began following the Formula, he drank coffee and snacked on donuts all morning. His complaints were poor concentration and trouble staying awake. Michael also began packing on the pounds, was too sluggish to exercise when work ended, and was desperate for a change. When he began following the Formula, he started his day with a 40-30-30 breakfast. He enjoyed drinking the Strawberry Smoothie on his drive to work and felt awake and much more creative. At 8:00 A.M. he ate a 40-30-30 snack. Michael had lunch at 11:00 A.M., and half of a 40-30-30 Nutrition Bar before he left work. The added energy that balanced, well-timed meals provided enabled him to drop by the corporate gym for 45 minutes each day before heading home. Michael claims he is performing better at work, with much more mental clarity and focus, as well as losing body fat. He also has new-found energy to spend with his three-year-old twin sons and his beautiful wife.

If you work unusual hours or extra long days, take the time to plan your Formula meals to suit your lifestyle.

29

DRINK APPROPRIATE AMOUNTS OF WATER

Water is one of the six essential nutrient classes your body requires for proper growth, maintenance, and repair. In fact, it is the most indispensable of the six groups necessary for survival. Water flows through every cell in your body, coursing through the arteries, capillaries, and veins. It is used for virtually all functions, including digestion, absorption, transporting nutrients, building tissues, and maintaining body temperature. All tissues contain water in varying amounts. Water makes up about three-fourths of muscle tissue, but only about one-fourth of body fat. Thus, lean individuals with a greater muscle mass to fat ratio have a greater percentage of body water than do obese individuals.

Most people don't drink enough water. Inadequate water consumption can cause heartburn, stomach cramps, low back pain, headaches, and fatigue. But if you drink adequate amounts of water, your body runs more smoothly, circulation is improved, digestion is enhanced, and your complexion is brightened.

The amount of water you require depends on your size and activity level. Rather than the standard eight 8-ounce glasses per day, use the

Personal Water Calculator to help you determine your individual water requirements:

Personal Water Calculator

1. Total body weight _____
2. Divide by 2 _____
3. Daily ounces of water per day _____

   My water requirements are_____

High-carbohydrate diets can elevate blood sugar and insulin levels. Insulin is a storage hormone and can cause your body to retain fluids. But a balanced diet can help to stabilize blood sugar and control insulin. You will no longer experience swollen feet or that bloated feeling from water retention.

Burning fat is also a very dehydrating process. Because toxins are stored in fat cells and fat is being burned for energy, toxins can be released in the bloodstream. Water becomes a critical vehicle to transport these toxins from your body. Because of this process, water becomes even more important when you are burning fat and losing weight.

Using the Personal Water Calculator, you can determine your individual water requirements and start drinking adequate amounts of this precious nutrient.

30

LIQUID MEALS WORK

Recent studies confirm that liquid meal replacements are a good way to lose weight and keep it off. Liquid meals help to remind us not to overeat, and following the personalized recipes found in *The Formula* will take the guesswork out of making a meal. When you prepare the Shake or Smoothie recipe correctly, you will be eating a perfect 40-30-30 Formula meal. Many of our clients know how to make their favorite Smoothies by heart.

Our friend Deb wakes up craving the O.J. Smoothie found in *The Formula*. She said it starts her day off perfectly and keeps her feeling great for the next four hours. When she deviates and has a different breakfast, she feels slightly off the whole morning.

So, the next time you're rushed or in the mood for something refreshing, blend up the delicious 40-30-30 Formula liquid meal on the following page. It really works!

FORMULA 40-30-30 FAT FLUSH
MEAL PLAN PERSONAL REQUIREMENTS*

Breakfast

KIDS' FAVORITE

O.J. Smoothie

	A	B	C	D	E
Orange juice	1/2 cup	1/2 cup	1/2 cup	1 cup	1 1/3 cups
Fresh orange, peeled	1/2 orange	1/2 orange	1 orange	1 orange	1 orange
Water and/or ice cubes	1/2 cup	1/2 cup	3/4 cup	3/4 cup	3/4 cup
Pure whey protein powder	13 grams	13 grams	20 grams	30 grams	30 grams
Almonds, sliced	1 1/3 tbsp.	1 1/3 tbsp.	2 1/3 tbsp.	3 tbsp.	3 2/3 tbsp.

DIRECTIONS: Combine all ingredients in a blender and process until smooth. *Note:* For more information on pure whey protein, please refer to Appendix C: Special Ingredients.

For more than 200 personalized meals and recipes, including the Formula 40-30-30 Fat Flush Meals, refer to our book *The Formula.*

*To know your A, B, C, D, or E Meal Plan Personal Requirements, refer to Appendix A: The Formula Meal Plan Selection Chart.

31

KEEP YOUR EYES OPEN
FOR NEW PRODUCTS

With millions of Americans turning away from the once popular high-carbohydrate, lowfat diet, the food industry is beginning to react. Food manufacturers have been scrambling to introduce protein-fortified cereals and reduce the amount of sugar and carbohydrate in many foods. It was only a few years ago that the hottest-selling food items were fat-free. But with new research pointing to elevated insulin as a direct link to obesity, diabetes, heart disease, stroke, high cholesterol, high blood pressure, gall bladder disease, and some types of cancer, balanced diets are becoming more prominent.

Your best choice for carbohydrate foods will always be fresh fruits and vegetables. They are predominantly low- to medium-glycemic foods that help control the release of insulin. Look for the new protein fortified tortillas, pastas, and breads made with whole grains and soy flour. They are less refined, contain more fiber and protein, and enter the bloodstream in a more controlled manner. When used as part of a balanced diet, blood sugar is stable and insulin is controlled. Sugary carbohydrate foods like soda, cookies, and candy should be avoided, as they enter the body quickly, elevate blood sugar, and trigger the release of insulin. Starchy carbohydrates like potatoes, white rice, pasta, and bread should be used in moderation, as they also can spike blood sugar and elevate insulin. Use red potatoes, sweet potatoes, and yams, brown or wild rice, and whole grain pasta, and breads instead. Manufacturers are finally beginning to cater to health-conscious individuals who read labels. Look for the new convenient protein sources like tuna in a pouch for added convenience when following the Formula.

Try the new lunch recipe on the following page that uses some of these new, protein-fortified "convenience" foods.

Lunch

High-Fiber Deli Wrap

	MEAL PLAN PERSONAL REQUIREMENTS*				
	A	B	C	D	E
Whole wheat flour tortilla, 6-inch diameter (La Tortilla Factory)	1	2	2	3	4
Lean sliced deli meat (turkey or chicken)	2 oz.	3½ oz.	3½ oz.	4 oz.	5 oz.
Swiss cheese, lowfat	1 oz.	1 oz.	1 oz.	1½ oz.	2 oz.
Avocado, medium	¼	⅓	⅓	⅓	½
Grapes, green or red	⅓ cup	½ cup	½ cup	½ cup	½ cup

DIRECTIONS: Place deli meat and cheese on tortilla. Top with sliced avocado and fold. Serve with fruit.

For more than 200 personalized meals and recipes, including the Formula 40-30-30 Fat Flush Meals, refer to our book *The Formula*.

*To know your A, B, C, D, or E Meal Plan Personal Requirements, refer to Appendix A: The Formula Meal Plan Selection Chart.

32

HAVE A CAESAR SALAD WEEK

f you've ever wanted a week of no-brainer dinners, try making Caesar salads every night. They are easy to prepare, delicious, and best of all, they are Formula 40-30-30 Fat Flush meals.

I received a phone call from Terri, a woman from Texas who was raving about her weight loss and thanking us for writing *The Formula.* She is a working mom with a husband and two teenage daughters. She began serving the meals to her family. Although she was never known as a great cook, her family began complimenting her newfound culinary skills. Their favorite dinner was the Chicken Caesar Salad with fruit. One of her daughters loved it so much she said, "Mom, I could eat this every night." Terri wanted to know if it was all right to have the salad nearly every night of the week. Although variety is the spice of life, as long as everyone likes it, there is nothing wrong with serving it often. After my conversation with Terri, we tried it for a week and found it to be very convenient.

Buy romaine lettuce in the large-size package at any of the big club stores. You can also stock up on the family-size portions of skinless, boneless chicken breasts, Parmesan cheese, olive oil, red wine vinegar, and fresh fruit. For variety, buy large salmon fillets, tuna steaks, jumbo shrimp, and lean steaks. Divide the protein into appropriate serving sizes, wrap, and freeze for later use. You can also use canned or packaged tuna, which requires no cooking.

If you love Caesar salads and could eat them every night, go ahead and make them often. For variety, rotate the protein and fruit you include.

Dinner

Grilled Salmon Caesar Salad

FORMULA 40-30-30 FAT FLUSH
MEAL PLAN PERSONAL REQUIREMENTS*

	A	B	C	D	E
Romaine lettuce, cleaned, dried, and torn	1/3 head	1/3 head	1/2 head	1/2 head	1/2 head
Grilled salmon, flaked	4 1/2 oz.	5 1/2 oz.	6 oz.	6 oz.	7 oz.
Caesar Dressing (recipe below)	2 1/4 tbsp.	2 1/2 tbsp.	3 tbsp.	3 tbsp.	3 tbsp.
Parmesan cheese, grated	1 tbsp.	1 tbsp.	1 1/2 tbsp.	1 1/2 tbsp.	2 1/2 tbsp.
Apple, medium	1/2	1	1	1	1
Grapes, green or red	3/4 cup	2/3 cup	3/4 cup	3/4 cup	1 1/4 cups

CAESAR DRESSING RECIPE:

2 tablespoons olive oil

2 tablespoons red wine vinegar

1 tablespoon lemon juice, fresh or bottled

1 small clove of garlic, pressed, or
   1 teaspoon garlic powder

1 teaspoon Worcestershire sauce

1 teaspoon anchovy paste (from tube)

1/2 teaspoon dry mustard powder

1/8 teaspoon pepper

1/8 teaspoon salt

RECIPE DIRECTIONS: Place all ingredients in a small jar and shake well.

DIRECTIONS: Toss romaine lettuce with Caesar Dressing. Top with flaked grilled salmon and sprinkle with Parmesan cheese. Serve with fresh fruit.

For more than 200 personalized meals and recipes, including the Formula 40-30-30 Fat Flush Meals, refer to our book *The Formula*.

*To know your A, B, C, D, or E Meal Plan Personal Requirements, refer to Appendix A: The Formula Meal Plan Selection Chart.

33

EXPERIMENT WITH RICE

◆

Rice can be a great source of carbohydrate to include as part of your 40-30-30 Formula meals. The nutritional values of rice can vary dramatically. White rice and instant white rice have been stripped of the majority of their nutritional value and have a high-glycemic rating. Brown, black, and wild rice still have their bran and germ attached, provide dietary fiber, and contain the original vitamins and minerals. These rice varieties have a lower glycemic rating. Although cooking times are longer, it is best to slightly undercook rice, (al dente) which lowers its glycemic response.

When including rice, limit it to approximately half of the total carbohydrates in the meal. Choose low-glycemic vegetables and fruits for the remaining carbohydrates. The combination of high-fiber, moderate-glycemic carbohydrates with low-glycemic carbohydrates along with protein and fat produces a meal that will stabilize blood sugar and control the release of insulin.

Try the great new Family Style Dinner on the next page.

	MEAL PLAN PERSONAL REQUIREMENTS*				
	A	B	C	D	E

Family Style Dinner
Stuffed Bell Pepper Cups

	A	B	C	D	E
Stuffed Bell Pepper Cups (recipe below)	1¼	1½	1¾	1¾	2
Mixed salad greens	2 cups	2 cups	2 cups	2 cups	3 cups
Oil and vinegar salad dressing	1 tbsp.	1 tbsp.	1½ tbsp.	1½ tbsp.	2 tbsp.
Black olives, medium	2	4	5	5	5
Apple, medium, sliced	½	¾	¾	¾	1

STUFFED BELL PEPPER CUPS RECIPE:

6 bell peppers, green or red, medium-large size

1 pound extra-lean ground beef, 5% fat

½ cup chopped onion

1 clove garlic, minced

½ teaspoon salt

¼ teaspoon pepper

1½ cups hot brown rice, cooked al dente

1½ cups canned tomatoes, diced, with liquid

1 egg, large

2 egg whites

1 teaspoon dried basil

1 teaspoon Worcestershire sauce

¼ cup cheddar cheese, ⅓ less fat, grated

RECIPE DIRECTIONS: Cut off the top ½" from peppers and remove seeds and membrane. Precook the peppers in salted boiling water for 5 minutes; drain. Cook ground beef with onion and garlic until meat is browned. Remove from heat and drain fat, if any. Add salt and pepper. Add tomatoes, rice, eggs, basil, and Worcestershire sauce. Fill the peppers with meat mixture and place upright in a baking dish. Sprinkle tops with cheese and bake uncovered at 375° for 25 minutes.

DIRECTIONS: Serve Bell Pepper Cups with olives, side salad, and apple.

For more than 200 personalized meals and recipes, including the Formula 40-30-30 Fat Flush Meals, refer to our book *The Formula*.

*To know your A, B, C, D, or E Meal Plan Personal Requirements, refer to Appendix A: The Formula Meal Plan Selection Chart.

34

PICTURE YOURSELF PERFECT

Whether your goal for following the Formula is to lose unwanted body fat and reach your ideal weight, to lose weight to improve a medical challenge, to slow the aging process, or for any other reason, picture yourself perfect with visualization. Visualization is a powerful tool you can use to help reach your goals. Athletes have been using this form of mental imagery for years.

If your goal is to lose weight, picture yourself at your ideal weight. By visualizing yourself lean, you begin programming your mind to prepare for that weight. It acts as a reminder to stay on track, continue to eat balanced meals, and maintain exercise. If your goal is to lower cholesterol or blood pressure while losing weight, draw a mental image of your cholesterol or blood pressure. While you are eating balanced meals or exercising, visualize your blood levels returning to normal and staying there. If your goal is to shape up to look and feel more youthful, imagine yourself younger and more fit. Envision the aging process slowing down and actually reversing. Visualize that the meals you eat are supplying supernutrients to your cells while your body builds and repairs itself.

Jeff, one of our clients and a competitive natural bodybuilder, used visualization to perfect his physique. He followed the Formula 40-30-30 Fat Flush to reach his weight class and get shredded. Each day, while posing, he would visualize himself with his perfect physique on stage winning the trophy.

Carol, a client following the Formula to lose weight and control diabetes, pictured herself healthy, fit, and completely in control of her blood sugar.

Mental imagery is a technique that can help you perform more confidently in every area of your life. If you practice visualization on a regular basis, it becomes easier to picture yourself perfect and reach your dietary health goals.

35

INCREASE ANTIOXIDANTS IN YOUR DIET WITH NUTRIENT-DENSE FRUITS

Nutrient-dense fruits are those that provide a high quantity of nutrients with a small quantity of calories. If one of your goals is to improve your health and reduce your risk of disease, choose carbohydrate sources that are nutrient-dense and high in the antioxidant phytochemicals. These plant chemicals fight against free-radical damage, protect your cells, and build your body's immune defenses.

Fortunately, the majority of nutrient-dense fruits also have low to medium glycemic ratings. When used as part of a balanced diet, they help stabilize blood sugar and control the hormone insulin. Typically, a greater amount of antioxidants are found in darker-colored fruits such as blueberries, raspberries, blackberries, strawberries, and purple grapes. They are also packed with vitamins, minerals, and fiber.

The next time you want to boost your supply of cell protectors, blend up one of the following delicious, new Formula 40-30-30 Fat Flush Breakfast Smoothies, rich in antioxidants.

Breakfast

KIDS' FAVORITE

Berry-Good for You Smoothie

	FORMULA 40-30-30 FAT FLUSH MEAL PLAN PERSONAL REQUIREMENTS*				
	A	B	C	D	E
Mixed berries, frozen (blueberries, blackberries, raspberries)	¾ cup	¾ cup	1⅓ cups	2 cups	2¼ cups
Water	¾ cup	¾ cup	1 cup	1½ cups	1½ cups
Pure whey protein powder	15 grams	15 grams	25 grams	35 grams	40 grams
Granulated fructose	1 tsp.	1 tsp.	1½ tsp.	1½ tsp.	1½ tsp.
Macadamia nuts, chopped	1 tbsp.	1 tbsp.	1¾ tbsp.	2 tbsp.	3 tbsp.

DIRECTIONS: Combine all ingredients in a blender and process until smooth. Granulated fructose can be found in health food stores. *Note:* For more information about pure whey protein, please refer to Appendix F: Special Ingredients.

Breakfast

Grape Smoothie

	FORMULA 40-30-30 FAT FLUSH MEAL PLAN PERSONAL REQUIREMENTS*				
	A	B	C	D	E
Purple seedless grapes, frozen	⅔ cup	⅔ cup	1 cup	1½ cups	1¾ cups
Water	½ cup	½ cup	¾ cup	1 cup	1¼ cups
Pure whey protein powder	15 grams	15 grams	25 grams	35 grams	40 grams
Granulated fructose	1 tsp.	1 tsp.	1½ tsp.	1½ tsp.	1½ tsp.
Macadamia nuts, chopped	1 tbsp.	1 tbsp.	1¾ tbsp.	2 tbsp.	3 tbsp.

DIRECTIONS: Combine all ingredients in a blender and process until smooth. Granulated fructose can be found in health food stores. *Note:* For more information about pure whey protein, please refer to Appendix C: Special Ingredients.

For more than 200 personalized meals and recipes, including the Formula 40-30-30 Fat Flush Meals, refer to our book *The Formula*.

*To know your A, B, C, D, or E Meal Plan Personal Requirements, refer to Appendix A: The Formula Meal Plan Selection Chart.

36

CEREAL
SOLUTIONS

We often hear people complain that they love the way they feel using the Formula, but they miss eating breakfast cereal. Well, you don't have to give up cereal if you know how to balance it. But you have a few choices to make. Because cereal is primarily carbohydrates, and high-glycemic at that, you need to decide what protein and fat to add to cereal to equal the 40-30-30 ratio. The protein and fat will slow the digestion of the cereal. This lowers the glycemic response of cereal, slowing its conversion into glucose, thereby helping to balance blood sugar and insulin.

First, decide if you want to add the protein and fat to the cereal. In that case, milk with added whey protein powder plus nuts is a great choice. If you prefer to have your cereal with milk and eat the additional protein and fat on the side, choose from lean Canadian bacon, sliced deli meats like turkey, chicken, or ham, eggs, or cottage cheese. You don't have to give up any of your favorite foods when following the Formula, just include them as part of your balanced diet.

The Formula provides many recipes for hot cereals and bran cereals. Here are a few new breakfast plans for you and your family to enjoy.

Breakfast
Cereal with Milk

	MEAL PLAN PERSONAL REQUIREMENTS*				
	A	B	C	D	E
Kellogg's Frosted Flakes	½ cup	½ cup	¾ cup	1 cup	1¼ cups
Milk, 1% lowfat	⅓ cup	⅓ cup	½ cup	½ cup	½ cup
Pure whey protein powder	15 grams	15 grams	20 grams	30 grams	35 grams
Macadamia nuts, chopped	2½ tsp.	2½ tsp.	1⅔ tbsp.	2 tbsp.	2⅔ tbsp.

DIRECTIONS: In a bowl, blend milk with whey protein powder. Add cereal and nuts. *Note:* For more information on pure whey protein, please refer to Appendix C: Special Ingredients.

Breakfast
Cereal with Eggs

	MEAL PLAN PERSONAL REQUIREMENTS*				
	A	B	C	D	E
Kellogg's Frosted Flakes	½ cup	½ cup	¾ cup	1 cup	1¼ cups
Milk, 1% lowfat	⅓ cup	⅓ cup	½ cup	¾ cup	¾ cup
Macadamia nuts, chopped	1 tsp.	1 tsp.	1 tbsp.	1⅓ tbsp.	1⅓ tbsp.
Eggs, whole	1	1	1	1	2
Eggs, whites only	2	2	4	6	6

DIRECTIONS: Scramble eggs in a nonstick skillet. Serve with a bowl of cereal topped with milk and nuts. *Note:* When feeding your hungry kids, serve the scrambled eggs first, then give them the cereal.

Breakfast
Bran Cereal with Milk

	MEAL PLAN PERSONAL REQUIREMENTS*				
	A	B	C	D	E
Kellogg's Cracklin' Bran	⅓ cup	⅓ cup	⅔ cup	¾ cup	1 cup
Milk, nonfat	⅓ cup	⅓ cup	½ cup	½ cup	⅔ cup
Pure whey protein powder	10 grams	10 grams	20 grams	30 grams	30 grams
Macadamia nuts, chopped	½ tbsp.	½ tbsp.	1 tbsp.	1 tbsp.	1½ tbsp.

DIRECTIONS: In a bowl, blend milk with whey protein powder. Add cereal and nuts.

For more than 200 personalized meals and recipes, including the Formula 40-30-30 Fat Flush Meals, refer to our book *The Formula*.

*To know your A, B, C, D, or E Meal Plan Personal Requirements, refer to Appendix A: The Formula Meal Plan Selection Chart.

37

DEVELOP BALANCED
MEALS FOR YOUR KIDS

We can't begin to tell you how often we have heard the desperate cry from parents about children who are picky eaters. Many children eat limited foods like spaghetti with butter, sugar-coated cereal, and mashed potatoes. We know it's easier to let them eat what they want rather than fight at the dinner table, but with childhood obesity and diabetes on the rise, you may want to reconsider that strategy.

It is important to begin discussing the significance of a balanced diet with children at any age. Teach your children which foods are carbohydrates, proteins, and fats, along with a simple explanation of the importance of each of these essential macronutrients:

- Carbohydrate foods provide fuel for your brain.
- Protein helps build strong muscles.
- Fat is important for hormone production to help you grow.

Encourage your children to help you prepare a balanced meal. Children love to get involved in family projects. Make a list of their favorite protein foods and post it in the kitchen. Have them review it often when you are preparing meals so they can choose from their favorites. Once they choose a protein food, it's easy to add the carbohydrates and fat. The following are sample lists from our nephew and niece, John and Katie.

SAMPLE PROTEIN FAVORITE FOODS LISTS

JOHN'S FAVORITE PROTEIN FOODS	KATIE'S FAVORITE PROTEIN FOODS
Chicken	Chicken
Eggs	Eggs
Steak	Steak
Lobster	Cheese
Cheese	Turkey (white meat)
Turkey	Yogurt with fruit
Clams	Jerky

This book, as well as *The Formula*, contains numerous recipes marked *Kids' Favorite*. We've heard from hundreds of parents who have tried these meals and are thrilled that their kids loved them. Try the following Top 10 Kids' Favorite meals on your picky eaters. The recipes can also be found in *The Formula*.

The Formula
Top 10 Kids' Favorite Meals

Breakfasts:

1. Strawberry Smoothie

2. One-Eyed Sandwich

Lunches:

3. Deli Meal 1

4. Grilled Ham and Cheese

Snacks:

5. Hard-Boiled Eggs and Apple

6. Chicken Fruit Skewers

Dinners:

7. Chicken Cheese Crisp (Mexican Pizza)

8. Macaroni and Cheese

9. Cheese Pizza

10. Taco Soup

TOP 10 KIDS' FAVORITE RECIPES
FORMULA 40-30-30 FAT FLUSH

Breakfast
Strawberry Smoothie

MEAL PLAN PERSONAL REQUIREMENTS*				
A	B	C	D	E
1 cup	1 cup	1⅔ cups	2 cups	2⅔ cups
½ cup	½ cup	¾ cup	1 cup	1 cup
13 grams	13 grams	20 grams	30 grams	30 grams
2 tsp.	2 tsp.	1 tbsp.	1⅔ tbsp.	1½ tbsp.
1⅓ tbsp.	1⅓ tbsp.	2⅓ tbsp.	3 tbsp.	3⅔ tbsp.

Ingredient labels:
- Strawberries, fresh or frozen
- Water, cold
- Pure whey protein powder
- Granulated fructose
- Almonds, sliced

DIRECTIONS: Combine all ingredients in a blender and process until smooth. Granulated fructose can be found in health food stores.

Breakfast
One-Eyed Sandwich

MEAL PLAN PERSONAL REQUIREMENTS*				
A	B	C	D	E
1 slice	1 slice	2 slices	3 slices	4 slices
½ tsp.	½ tsp.	½ tsp.	1 tsp.	1 tsp.
1	1	2	2	3
2	2	2	4	4
½	½	¾	1	1

Ingredient labels:
- Bread, whole grain
- Whipped butter
- Eggs, whole
- Eggs, whites only
- Orange, medium, quartered

DIRECTIONS: Remove and discard a 3-inch diameter circle from the center of bread slices. Lightly butter the remaining edges and place in a hot, nonstick pan. Break eggs and whites in center and cook until set. Turn to brown both sides. Salt and pepper to taste. Serve with orange slices.

Lunch
Deli Meal 1

	A	B	C	D	E
Sliced deli meat (turkey, chicken, lean ham, or beef)	2½ oz.	3 oz.	3 oz.	4 oz.	6 oz.
Sliced Swiss cheese, lowfat	1 oz.	2 oz.	2 oz.	2½ oz.	3 oz.
Apple or pear	1 medium	1 large	1 large	1 medium + 1 large	2 large

MEAL PLAN PERSONAL REQUIREMENTS*

DIRECTIONS: In a grocery store deli, order your specific amount of sliced deli meat and cheese and grab an apple or pear in the produce department.

MEAL PLAN PERSONAL REQUIREMENTS*

Lunch
Grilled Ham and Cheese

	A	B	C	D	E
Bread, reduced-calorie, wheat or white	2 slices	3 slices	3 slices	4 slices	5 slices
Whipped butter	2 tsp.	1 tbsp.	1 tbsp.	1⅓ tbsp.	1½ tbsp.
Ham, extra-lean deli-style	1½ oz.	2½ oz.	2½ oz.	3 oz.	4 oz.
Swiss cheese, lowfat	1 oz.	1½ oz.	1½ oz.	2 oz.	2½ oz.
Dill pickle	1	1	1	1	1
Peach, medium	½	1	1	1	1

DIRECTIONS: Grill a lightly buttered ham and cheese sandwich until golden brown on both sides. Serve with dill pickle and fresh peach.

Snack
Hard-Boiled Eggs and Apple

	A	B	C	D	E
Eggs, whole	1	1	1	1	2
Egg whites	2	2	2	2	4
Apple, medium, sliced	1	1	1	1	2

MEAL PLAN PERSONAL REQUIREMENTS*

DIRECTIONS: Hard-boil eggs. Peel cooled eggs and discard the appropriate number of yolks. Add salt and pepper to taste and serve with apple slices.

FORMULA 40-30-30 FAT FLUSH
MEAL PLAN PERSONAL REQUIREMENTS*

Snack
Chicken Fruit Skewers

	A	B	C	D	E
Chicken breast, cooked, cooled, and cubed	2 oz.	2 oz.	2 oz.	2 oz.	4 oz.
Black olives, large	3	3	3	3	6
Grapes, red	10	10	10	10	20
Apple, medium, cored and cubed	½	½	½	½	1

DIRECTIONS: Alternate chicken, olives, grapes, and apple chunks on wooden skewers.

MEAL PLAN PERSONAL REQUIREMENTS*

Dinner
Chicken Cheese Crisp (Mexican Pizza)

	A	B	C	D	E
Flour tortillas, 7- to 8-inch diameter	2	2	2½	2½	3
Jalapeño cheese, shredded	2½ tbsp.	2½ tbsp.	3 tbsp.	3 tbsp.	4 tbsp.
Cheddar cheese, 50% reduced fat, shredded	2 tbsp.	2 tbsp.	2½ tbsp.	2½ tbsp.	3 tbsp.
Green chilies, canned or fresh, diced	2 tbsp.	2 tbsp.	2½ tbsp.	2½ tbsp.	3 tbsp.
Cooked chicken breast, cubed	2½ oz.	3 oz.	3½ oz.	3½ oz.	4½ oz.
Black olives, large	4	6	6	6	6

DIRECTIONS: Preheat oven to 400°F. Place tortillas on a baking sheet, spray lightly with olive oil spray, and bake until crisp. Top tortilla with jalapeño and cheddar cheese, chilies, chicken, and sliced olives. Return to oven for 10–15 minutes until cheese melts and begins to brown.

MEAL PLAN PERSONAL REQUIREMENTS*

Dinner
Macaroni and Cheese with Chicken Dinner

	A	B	C	D	E
Macaroni and Cheese (recipe below)	¾ cup	1 cup	1¼ cup	1¼ cup	1½ cup
Chicken breast (cooked amount)	2½ oz.	2½ oz.	3 oz.	3 oz.	4 oz.
Green beans, fresh or canned	¾ cup	1 cup	1 cup	1 cup	1½ cup
Peach, fresh, medium, or ½ cup canned, drained	1	1	1	1	1

MACARONI AND CHEESE RECIPE:

3 cups elbow macaroni, cooked

3 tablespoons olive oil

2 tablespoons flour

½ teaspoon salt

⅛ teaspoon pepper

2 cups milk, 1% lowfat

8 ounces cheddar cheese, lowfat

RECIPE DIRECTIONS: Preheat oven to 350°F. In a saucepan, heat oil and blend in flour, salt, and pepper. Add milk and stir until thick and bubbly. Add cheese chunks until melted. Add cooked macaroni and mix thoroughly. Place in a casserole dish and bake at 350° for 35 minutes or until heated through and lightly browned.

DIRECTIONS: Serve Macaroni and Cheese with chicken, green beans, and peach.

Dinner

Cheese Pizza

	MEAL PLAN PERSONAL REQUIREMENTS*				
	A	B	C	D	E
Flour tortillas, 7- to 8-inch diameter	1⅔	2	2	2	2½
Pizza sauce	3 tbsp.	3 tbsp.	4 tbsp.	4 tbsp.	6 tbsp.
Mozzarella cheese, part-skim, shredded	½ cup	½ cup	½ cup	½ cup	⅔ cup
Mozzarella cheese, nonfat, shredded	⅓ cup	⅓ cup	½ cup	½ cup	⅔ cup

DIRECTIONS: Preheat oven to 400°F. Place tortillas on a baking sheet and bake until crisp. Spread tortilla with pizza sauce and top with cheese. Return to oven for 10–15 minutes until cheese melts and begins to brown.

Dinner

Taco Soup Dinner

	MEAL PLAN PERSONAL REQUIREMENTS*				
	A	B	C	D	E
Taco Soup (recipe below)	1¾ cup	2 cups	2½ cups	2½ cups	3¼ cups
Sour cream, lowfat	2 tbsp.	2 tbsp.	3 tbsp.	3 tbsp.	3½ tbsp.
Cheddar cheese, full-fat, shredded	1 tbsp.	1 tbsp.	2 tbsp.	2 tbsp.	3 tbsp.
Corn taco shell, small, crumbled	1	1	2	2	3

TACO SOUP RECIPE:

1½ pounds extra-lean ground sirloin

1 tablespoon olive oil

1 cup diced onion

1 clove minced garlic

28-ounce canned tomatoes, diced, with juice

15-ounce canned tomato sauce

15¼-ounce canned black beans, with juice

8¾-ounce canned corn, with juice

1-ounce package of taco seasoning mix

RECIPE DIRECTIONS: In a medium, heavy pot, heat oil. Add the ground sirloin and brown. Add onion and garlic and cook for 5 minutes. Add canned tomatoes, tomato sauce, beans, corn, and taco seasoning mix. Cook 30 minutes longer.

DIRECTIONS: In a bowl, serve taco soup topped with sour cream, cheese, and crumbled taco shell.

For more than 200 personalized meals and recipes, including the Formula 40-30-30 Fat Flush Meals, refer to our book *The Formula*.

*To know your A, B, C, D, or E Meal Plan Personal Requirements, refer to Appendix A: The Formula Meal Plan Selection Chart.

38

IGNITE FAT LOSS WITH TWO-A-DAY WORKOUTS

I f you are trying to burn fat even faster for a special event or you've set a goal weight and want to do everything possible to reach it, start increasing your workouts to double days. Exercise is a powerful adjunct to the Formula. The Formula is a dietary lifestyle that actually helps set up your body to maximize its natural fat-burning potential. Exercise can dramatically improve your access to stored body fat. It not only makes you feel better, healthier, and more fit, but exercise also lowers insulin (the fat-storing hormone) and increases glucagon and human growth hormone (the fat-burning and muscle-building hormones). Exercise increases the activity of fat-burning enzymes and helps reduce harmful blood fats.

We've worked with thousands of athletes through the years and have seen the power of exercise with the Formula. But some of the most impressive fat loss happens when individuals follow the Formula and exercise twice per day.

One of our clients, a housewife and mother of two, began using our program in May 1999. At first, she didn't make time for exercise, but lost 10 pounds in 2½ weeks. We encouraged her to start walking each morning with her one-year-old son. She loaded up the stroller and walked for 45 to

60 minutes. In the next two weeks, she had lost another 8 pounds and was feeling and looking great. Her goal was to lose another 20 pounds by the end of summer, but she had her 10-year class reunion to attend the first of August and was determined to do everything possible to reach that goal. She was doing great following her personalized plan but wanted to know what else she could do to get even faster results. After reviewing her meal plans and morning walking schedule, we suggested she follow the Formula 40-30-30 Fat Flush meals exclusively and add an extra workout in the evening. We recommended a workout that included additional cardiovascular training as well as strength training and stretching.

She bought a yoga tape and built up to 45 minutes each night after dinner. She found it to be a great cardiovascular workout, and it provided strength and resistance as well as stretching. She was amazed at how relaxed it made her feel and how soundly she slept. Best of all, she lost the extra 20 pounds and looked great in a new dress at the reunion.

If you want to ignite your fat loss, try the following formula:

1. Follow the Formula 40-30-30 Fat Flush meal plans exclusively. Make sure you choose the correct plan for your size and activity level.
2. Work out twice per day. Do a morning and evening workout that includes cardiovascular training, strength or resistance training, and stretching.

Note: Be sure to drink plenty of water to prevent dehydration before and after exercise and always check with your health care professional before starting any exercise or nutrition program.

39

DON'T
UNDEREAT

A common mistake people make when following the Formula is to not eat enough food. This may fly in the face of everything you've heard about losing weight. We know you've heard the saying, "To lose weight you must reduce calories," but very-low-calorie diets can be dangerous. They can be too low in essential fats and protein and can cause hormonal imbalances and muscle loss.

The Formula is a balanced nutrition program, personalized for your specific requirements. Choosing the correct size meal plan is critical. A simple way to look at it is that you need adequate nutrients and calories to maintain your lean muscle mass. The more muscle mass you have, the more calories your body requires to maintain it. Excess body fat requires zero calories.

Many clients have actually slowed their fat loss by eating less food than recommended. One client weighed 202 pounds when she began following the Formula. Using the C plan she lost 12 pounds in the first two weeks. After four weeks, her weight loss had slowed down, her energy levels were low, and she complained of hunger between meals. Her problem was evident when she mentioned that she had dropped to the A plan to speed up her results. We explained that eating fewer calories slowed her metabolism, fat loss, and energy level, and increased hunger. She was back on track at her next meal. When her weight dropped to 180 pounds, she switched to the B plan and continued losing body fat while avoiding plateaus or energy slumps.

Be sure you are following the correct size plan for your sex, weight, and activity level.

40

TRY A BALANCED POPCORN SNACK

Popcorn has always been thought of as a great diet food because it's low in calories and fat. But new research on its glycemic rating has caused us to reconsider. The glycemic index rating is a measure of how fast carbohydrate foods break down into glucose and enter the bloodstream. A rapid rise in blood sugar stimulates the release of insulin to lower it.

The glycemic rating of a carbohydrate food is based on that food when eaten alone. When carbohydrate foods are eaten with protein and fat, the overall effect of that meal will be lower. Protein and fat slow the digestion of the meal so that carbohydrates are converted into glucose more slowly, thereby maintaining steady blood sugar levels and controlling the release of insulin.

Popcorn is a high-glycemic food and is typically eaten alone or with a lot of added fat from butter. But if you want to eat popcorn, include some protein and a little fat with it. You can dramatically change the overall glycemic response, slow its digestion, and have tighter control of blood glucose levels.

Try this recipe the next time you want a balanced popcorn snack.

Cheese Popcorn Snack

¼ cup popcorn, uncooked (equals 3 cups popped)

½ tablespoon olive oil

3 tablespoons Parmesan cheese, grated

13 grams pure whey protein powder

Spray olive oil

Salt

DIRECTIONS: Heat olive oil in a heavy pan until hot. Add popcorn and shake until completely popped. Blend Parmesan cheese, whey protein powder, and a dash of salt in a small cup. Place popcorn in a large bowl and spray lightly with olive oil spray and toss with the cheese mixture to coat. Spray once again with olive oil spray and toss again. *Note:* For more information on pure whey protein, please refer to the Appendix at the back of the book. *Note:* If air-popped corn is used, drizzle ½ teaspoon of olive oil over popcorn before coating with cheese mixture.

Per Serving: Grams=C-26g; P-20g; F-10g.

41

LEARN HOW TO MAKE SUBSTITUTIONS

What if you don't like a particular food in your personalized meal planner? Simply learn how to make easy substitutions. The Formula is the world's most complete personalized 40-30-30 nutrition program. We act as your very own personal nutrition coaches and show you exactly what to eat. Based on your sex, weight, and activity levels, you are provided with a complete personalized meal planner. These planners provide you with more than 200 personalized 40-30-30 meals and recipes. But, if a recipe or meal calls for a food you don't like, don't freak out or give up. Simply don't eat that food and substitute something that you do like. The Formula and 40-30-30 nutrition are all about balance. There are no bad or forbidden foods; any food can be used as long as it is part of a balanced meal or snack.

Here are a few basic guidelines to help you to learn how to substitute different foods that are used in a meal or recipe found in *The Formula*:

- *Carbohydrate substitutions:* Substitute equal amounts of any vegetable for equal amounts of any other vegetable, any fruit for fruit, and any starch for starch as long as they contain approximately the same glycemic rating.

- *Protein substitutions:* Substitute equal amounts of any lowfat protein for equal amounts of any other lowfat protein. Vegetarians can substitute any objectionable protein with equal amounts of lowfat vegetarian protein, as long as it is low in carbohydrate and fat, such as lowfat tofu or tempeh.

- *Fat substitutions:* Substitute equal amounts of any oil for any other oil, any nut for any other nut, or any lowfat cheese for another lowfat cheese. You can also substitute equal amounts of full-fat mayonnaise with avocado.

So, if you come across a certain food that you don't like, simply learn how to make these easy substitutions. Don't freak out, just substitute.

42

COOK LARGE PORTIONS

When you find a meal or recipe that you and your family really enjoy, make a double batch and freeze the leftovers. One of our favorite Family Style meals is the Vegetable Chili Dinner recipe found in *The Formula*. We make two pots at a time, let them cool, and portion out the correct serving size—2 cups for Joyce, 2½ cups for Gene—and freeze it in freezer bags. When we don't feel like cooking, we just pull out the bags and heat and eat in less than 15 minutes.

We encourage the use of Family Style meals even if you cook only for yourself. The leftovers make great frozen meals in minutes.

	FORMULA 40-30-30 FAT FLUSH MEAL PLAN PERSONAL REQUIREMENTS*				
Dinner	A	B	C	D	E

KIDS' FAVORITE / *Family Style*

Vegetable Chili

	A	B	C	D	E
Vegetable Chili	1½ cups	1¾ cups	2 cups	2 cups	3 cups
Apple, medium	1	1	1	1	1

VEGETABLE CHILI RECIPE:

½ pound chicken breast, cubed

1 pound extra-lean ground beef or chopped sirloin

3 stalks celery, chopped

1 cup chopped red or green pepper

1 cup chopped onion

1½ cups chopped mushrooms

½ cup diced fresh parsley

1 package chili seasoning mix

28-ounce can crushed tomatoes with juice

15-ounce can tomato sauce

6-ounce can tomato paste

6-ounce can water

RECIPE DIRECTIONS: Brown chicken and beef in a large Dutch oven or soup pot. Add celery, peppers, onions, mushrooms, and parsley. Cook until vegetables begin to soften. Add chili seasoning mix, tomatoes, tomato sauce, tomato paste, and water. Mix well and simmer for at least 1 hour. If you like your chili spicy, add ½ to 1 teaspoon crushed red pepper flakes.

DIRECTIONS: Serve chili with fresh apple slices.

For more than 200 personalized meals and recipes, including the Formula 40-30-30 Fat Flush Meals, refer to our book *The Formula*.

*To know your A, B, C, D, or E Meal Plan Personal Requirements, refer to Appendix A: The Formula Meal Plan Selection Chart.

43

SLOW THE AGING PROCESS

What's one thing that we never think of as kids but always think of as adults? No, not that. We're referring to aging. We all have hormones in our bodies that either speed up or slow down the aging process. Research is pointing to a nutrient-dense, balanced diet as our best defense against aging.

Studies on longevity point out that excess calories and insulin increase free-radical damage that can accelerate aging. Animal studies have shown that those who were fed the fewest amount of calories but with the greatest amount of nutrients doubled their lifespan. Therefore, a nutrient-dense, reduced-calorie diet becomes a powerful tool available to all of us to produce a longer, more functional life while reducing our risk of disease.

Although none of us can live forever, we can use balanced nutrition to improve the chemical reactions in our body to slow the aging process. Anti-aging should not be thought of as just living longer—but as living better.

Try this delicious Asparagus Chicken Quiche meal for a light dinner some night. It is a nutrient-dense meal that is naturally low in calories. It is a great source of easy-to-digest, high-quality protein that is easy to chew, making it an excellent meal for many seniors.

Time may go by quickly, but slowing the aging process is something we can begin to control with a balanced Formula diet.

Dinner
Family Style
Asparagus Chicken Quiche

	MEAL PLAN PERSONAL REQUIREMENTS*				
	A	B	C	D	E
Asparagus Chicken Quiche (recipe below)	2 slices	2½ slices	3 slices	3 slices	3½ slices
Tomatoes, large, sliced	2 slices	2 slices	2 slices	2 slices	3 slices
Mixed berries (strawberries and blueberries)	¾ cup	¾ cup	¾ cup	¾ cup	1 cup

CRUST RECIPE:

Prepare crust:

1 cup whole wheat flour

½ teaspoon salt

2 tablespoons canola oil

¼ cup + 1 tablespoon nonfat milk

CRUST DIRECTIONS (*Note:* You can also use a prepared pie crust.): In a bowl, blend flour and salt. Blend oil and milk and pour over dry ingredients. Stir with a fork until blended. Pat dough evenly over the bottom and sides of a deep 9-inch pie pan. Brush crust with one beaten egg yolk and prebake crust in 425° oven for 3–4 minutes to set egg glaze. Remove from oven and fill with Quiche mixture. Turn oven down to 375°.

ASPARAGUS CHICKEN QUICHE RECIPE:

2 large eggs

4 egg whites

⅔ cup nonfat milk

½ teaspoon salt

¼ teaspoon ground black pepper

⅔ cup precooked or canned asparagus, 2-inch pieces

2 cups cooked chicken, cubed

QUICHE DIRECTIONS: Beat eggs, whites, milk, salt, and pepper. In the bottom of the pie crust, place cooked chicken and asparagus. Top with egg mixture. Bake in 375°F oven until filling is browned and set (25–35 minutes). Let sit for 10 minutes before cutting into 8 even slices.

DIRECTIONS: Have Quiche with tomatoes and mixed berries.

For more than 200 personalized meals and recipes, including the Formula 40-30-30 Fat Flush Meals, refer to our book *The Formula*.

*To know your A, B, C, D, or E Meal Plan Personal Requirements, refer to Appendix A: The Formula Meal Plan Selection Chart.

44

HAVE A COOK-OFF DAY

If you lead a busy lifestyle and find it difficult at times to prepare meals, plan ahead by having a couple of cook-off days a month. These are days you take the time to prepare several of our Family-Size Meals found in this book and *The Formula*. Divide them into your portion requirements and freeze them. Precooked Chicken Breast (for Chicken Caesar Salad), Lasagna, Chicken Vegetable or Beef Barley Soup, Jambalaya, Taco Soup, Vegetable Chili, and Shredded Chicken are quick to thaw and reheat for lightning-fast meals.

One of our favorite meals is the Shredded Chicken recipe found in our book *The Formula*. We usually make two pots at the same time, one with chicken and one with beef. Later in the day, after they cool, simply shred the meat (pull it apart with forks), portion it into small plastic bags, and freeze. We use it for burritos or in a taco salad or omelettes.

So, plan a cook-off day. It can make preparing healthy, fat-burning meals deliciously easy.

Dinner

KIDS' FAVORITE
Shredded Chicken Burritos

	MEAL PLAN PERSONAL REQUIREMENTS*				
	A	B	C	D	E
Flour tortilla, 7- to 8-inch diameter	1½	1¾	2	2	2½
Sour cream, full-fat	2 tbsp.	2⅓ tbsp.	2¾ tbsp.	2¾ tbsp.	3 tbsp.
Refried beans, canned	1½ tbsp.	2 tbsp.	2 tbsp.	2 tbsp.	2½ tbsp.
Shredded Chicken (recipe below)	⅔ cup	⅔ cup	¾ cup	¾ cup	1 cup
Lettuce, shredded	¼ cup	¼ cup	⅓ cup	⅓ cup	⅓ cup
Tomato, chopped	¼ cup	¼ cup	⅓ cup	⅓ cup	⅓ cup
Salsa	3 tbsp.	3 tbsp.	3 tbsp.	3 tbsp.	3 tbsp.

SHREDDED CHICKEN RECIPE:

2 pounds boneless chicken, breast meat only

¼ cup water

3 tablespoons red wine vinegar

1½ cups chicken broth

2 tablespoons chili powder

1 teaspoon ground cumin

RECIPE DIRECTIONS: Place chicken breasts in a 5- to 6-quart pot with water and cook over medium heat for 30 minutes. Uncover and cook until liquid evaporates and chicken begins to brown. In a bowl, blend vinegar, chicken broth, chili powder, and cumin. Add to meat and continue cooking over medium heat until chicken is very tender and pulls apart easily (about 1 hour). Let chicken cool; shred it with two forks. Mix with remaining pan juices.

DIRECTIONS: Place sour cream, refried beans, and shredded chicken mixture on warmed flour tortilla. Top with lettuce, tomato, and salsa. Fold burrito-style.

For more than 200 personalized meals and recipes, including the Formula 40-30-30 Fat Flush Meals, refer to our book *The Formula*.

*To know your A, B, C, D, or E Meal Plan Personal Requirements, refer to Appendix A: The Formula Meal Plan Selection Chart.

45

HAVE A FEW BITES OF PROTEIN FIRST

I f you are extra sensitive to carbohydrates, especially high- and very-high-glycemic carbohydrate foods, you may want to get in the habit of eating several bites of protein in your meal before any of the carbohydrates. Protein and fat in a meal digest more slowly than carbohydrates. By eating a few bites of protein first, you are able to slow the digestion of the entire meal to more tightly control blood sugar levels.

Here are some examples:

- If you are eating eggs with toast and fruit for breakfast, eat 3 to 4 bites of egg before eating any toast or fruit.
- If you are eating tuna salad with fruit for lunch, eat several bites of the tuna salad before you eat any of the fruit.
- If you are are eating grilled salmon with red potatoes, asparagus, and a salad for dinner, have several bites of the salmon and salad before eating the potatoes.

It's not necessary to eat all of your protein first, then move on to the rest of the meal. One-pot meals like soups, chili, casseroles, Formula

Smoothies and Shakes, and 40-30-30 Nutrition Bars have the carbohydrate, protein, and fat combined, making it impossible to eat the protein first. Don't worry: Those meals are well-blended and provide the proper 40-30-30 ratio in every bite.

The main point is to avoid eating mostly carbohydrates first, then protein. This is a great tip to use when trying to feed young children balanced meals. Children tend to eat carbohydrates first and leave the protein. If you are having trouble getting your youngsters to eat all of their meal in the proper balance, serve the protein first. When children are hungry, they eat the first thing you give them. Our nephew used to eat all the carbohydrates and play with the protein. Now, his mother serves him scrambled eggs first, followed by peaches and toast. It was a simple solution to make sure he was getting adequate protein.

Here's a great new Family Style soup recipe. Serve it with a side salad for a delicious, balanced Formula dinner.

Dinner
Family Style
Split Pea and Ham Soup

	MEAL PLAN PERSONAL REQUIREMENTS*				
	A	B	C	D	E
Soup (recipe below)	1½ cups	1¾ cups	2 cups	2 cups	2⅓ cups
Mixed salad greens	2 cups	2 cups	2½ cups	2½ cups	3 cups
Oil and vinegar salad dressing	1½ tbsp.	1½ tbsp.	1¾ tbsp.	1¾ tbsp.	2 tbsp.

SPLIT PEA AND HAM SOUP RECIPE:

2 cups dried peas

4 cups water

3 cups chicken broth

1 bay leaf

½ teaspoon dry mustard

½ teaspoon dried thyme

½ teaspoon dried rosemary

1 teaspoon dried basil

1 teaspoon salt

¼ teaspoon ground black pepper

2 tablespoons olive oil

3 cloves garlic, diced

1 cup carrots, diced

1 cup celery, diced

1 cup onion, diced

½ cup red bell pepper, diced

1½ pounds extra-lean ham steak (sliced ½-inch thick), cut into ½-inch cubes

1 cup light or dark beer

RECIPE DIRECTIONS: Rinse split peas in a colander. In a large pot, place peas, water, and broth. Bring to a boil, remove foam, and reduce to a simmer. Add seasonings (next 7 ingredients) and cook on low simmer for 1 hour. Heat olive oil in a sauté pan and cook garlic, carrots, celery, onion, and bell pepper until soft. Add sautéed vegetables to the peas. *Optional:* You can puree the vegetables and peas at this point with a hand blender for a creamier texture. Add beer and ham and cook for 20–30 minutes.

DIRECTIONS: Serve soup with dinner salad and dressing.

For more than 200 personalized meals and recipes, including the Formula 40-30-30 Fat Flush Meals, refer to our book *The Formula*.

*To know your A, B, C, D, or E Meal Plan Personal Requirements, refer to Appendix A: The Formula Meal Plan Selection Chart.

46

GET RID OF
JUNK FOOD

◆

Some of the best advice we've given through the years has also been the simplest: Get rid of all junk food. When clients begin following the Formula, they are generally focused on and excited about their results. As the pounds begin melting off, energy levels improve and they begin looking better and feeling great. But there have been times when trouble sets in.

One client who lost 25 pounds began to complain that she hit a plateau. After questioning her to find out what she was doing differently, we discovered that she was nibbling on cookies and crackers she kept in the house for her children's lunches. We asked her a few questions: "Do you believe the Formula is the most healthy dietary plan you've ever followed?" She answered yes. "Then why are you feeding your children a high-carbohydrate, high-sugar diet?" Her response was that it was what she had always done in the past.

We suggested she replace the cookies and crackers with balanced 40-30-30 Formula lunches instead. With that, she got rid of the junk food in her cabinets, including sugary cereals, cookies, candy, crackers, and chips. By removing the temptations completely, the entire family began to benefit by following the Formula.

When high-carbohydrate foods in your cabinets or refrigerator tempt you, get rid of them. It's a lot easier to follow the Formula when you fill your shelves with healthy, nutrient-dense foods.

47

THE FORMULA IS YOUR KEY TO SUPERHEALTH

Although the Formula is primarily thought of as a personalized dietary plan for losing unwanted body fat, the health benefits of a balanced diet are enormous. Research is beginning to point to high blood sugar and excess insulin as the culprit in many diseases. Poorly balanced diets stimulate negative hormonal reactions in the body that weaken the immune system, increasing susceptibility to illness and disease. If a balanced diet can stabilize blood sugar levels, it will ultimately give you the power to control excess insulin.

Lowering excess insulin can decrease your risk of hypoglycemia, obesity, diabetes, high blood pressure, high cholesterol, and certain types of cancer. Stabilizing blood sugar can improve sleep patterns, brain concentration and clarity, moods and behavior, and balance and stabilize hormonal reactions.

The Formula provides a balanced nutrition solution for a healthy life. It can give you the peace of mind that you do have the power to reduce your likelihood of disease. Now you can not only live longer and healthier—with the Formula, you can have superhealth.

48

DON'T SKIP BREAKFAST

◆

You've always heard that breakfast is the most important meal of the day. But why? We've found that when we take the time to explain why, people are more likely to make time for this all-important meal.

If you finish eating dinner at 7:30 P.M., sleep through the night, and wake up at 7:30 A.M., you've actually just fasted for 12 hours. While you were sleeping, your body was working to repair itself. The food you ate at your evening meal supplies the essential nutrients: glucose, amino acids, fatty acids, vitamins, minerals, and water. During sleep, these essential nutrients are used for energy to build and repair more than 50,000 different body proteins, such as those in hair, skin, nails, hormones, enzymes, blood, neurotransmitters, and cells. When you wake, it is critical to replenish these essential nutrients by once again eating a balanced meal.

If you skip breakfast, blood sugar levels can begin to dip and energy level and mental clarity can suffer. If you don't eat until noon, the lack of essential nutrients can begin to affect your protein stores. Your body can be forced to rob from existing body proteins to supply the necessary essential nutrients your bloodstream is lacking. If you grab a quick cup of coffee and a sweet roll, blood sugar can spike, stimulating the release of insulin to lower it. The coffee and sweet roll lack essential nutrients and can lead to energy slumps, moodiness, and mental dullness.

But, by eating a balanced meal within one hour after waking, you can stabilize blood sugar and control insulin. The carbohydrate, protein, and fat provide a fresh supply of essential nutrients needed to build body proteins and hormones that get you through the morning with energy to spare, along with better clarity and focus.

So, don't miss breakfast. It really is the most important meal of the day. Think of it as your first opportunity to program your body to burn fat as your primary source of fuel and to supply the nutrients you need to look and feel great.

Here's a delicious, nutrient-packed recipe and a great way to "break the fast" any morning.

Breakfast
Formula Benedict

	MEAL PLAN PERSONAL REQUIREMENTS*				
	A	B	C	D	E
English muffin, toasted	½	½	1	1	1½
Canadian bacon, 98% fat-free	2 oz.	2 oz.	2½ oz.	4 oz.	4 oz.
Poached eggs, large	1	1	2	2	2½
Easy Hollandaise Sauce (recipe below)	1 tbsp.	1 tbsp.	1¼ tbsp.	2 tbsp.	3 tbsp.
Strawberries	¾ cup	¾ cup	½ cup	1½ cups	1 cup

EASY HOLLANDAISE SAUCE RECIPE:

2 tablespoons light sour cream
2 tablespoons lowfat mayonnaise
1 teaspoon brown mustard
1 teaspoon lemon juice, fresh
1 tablespoon lowfat milk
Salt and pepper to taste

RECIPE DIRECTIONS: Blend all ingredients in a small sauce pan. Cook and stir over low heat until warm. Makes enough for several servings.

DIRECTIONS: Top toasted English muffin with warmed Canadian bacon and well drained poached egg and drizzle with Easy Hollandaise Sauce. Serve with sliced strawberries.

For more than 200 personalized meals and recipes, including the Formula 40-30-30 Fat Flush Meals, refer to our book *The Formula*.

*To know your A, B, C, D, or E Meal Plan Personal Requirements, refer to Appendix A: The Formula Meal Plan Selection Chart.

49

REDUCE THE GLYCEMIC
EFFECT OF STARCHY FOODS

The way you cook starchy foods like rice and pasta can change the glycemic effect of those foods. If you cook rice and pasta until tender, they digest and convert into glucose rather quickly. The faster the rise in glucose, the faster the rise in insulin.

But, if you remember to slightly undercook rice and pasta (al dente) and always eat them with protein and fat, you can lower their glycemic response and better control blood sugar and insulin levels. Use a timer when cooking pasta for best results.

PASTA COOKING TIMES

Firm (al dente)	7–9 minutes
Medium	11 minutes
Well-done	12 minutes

MEAL PLAN PERSONAL REQUIREMENTS*

Dinner
Family Style

Tuna Mac Casserole Dinner

	A	B	C	D	E
Tuna Mac Casserole (recipe below)	2 slices	2⅓ slices	2⅔ slices	2⅔ slices	3⅓ slice
Mixed salad greens	2 cups	2 cups	2 cups	2 cups	2 cups
Olive oil and vinegar dressing	1 tbsp.	1 tbsp.	1 tbsp.	1 tbsp.	1 tbsp.
Strawberries, sliced	¾ cup	¾ cup	1 cup	1 cup	1 cup

TUNA MAC CASSEROLE RECIPE:

3 cups cooked whole wheat macaroni

2 tablespoons olive oil

1½ cups mushrooms, sliced

1½ cups broccoli, chopped

½ cup red bell pepper, diced

½ cup onions, diced

¼ cup flour

2½ cups milk, 1% lowfat

¾ cup cheddar cheese, ⅓ less fat

14 ounces albacore tuna

RECIPE DIRECTIONS: Cook whole wheat macaroni for 7 minutes (al dente). Do not overcook. Drain and set aside. Heat olive oil in a large sauté pan. Add mushrooms, broccoli, bell pepper, and onions and cook until just tender. Stir in flour and cook for 1 minute. Add milk, stirring until thick. Spray a large casserole dish (15x10x2) with olive oil. Pour in cooked macaroni. Add cheese and flaked tuna and top with vegetable sauce. Sprinkle with salt and pepper to taste. Bake at 375° for 25 minutes or until bubbly. Cut into 12 equal slices.

DIRECTIONS: Serve Tuna Mac Casserole with salad, dressing, and fruit.

For more than 200 personalized meals and recipes, including the Formula 40-30-30 Fat Flush Meals, refer to our book *The Formula*.

*To know your A, B, C, D, or E Meal Plan Personal Requirements, refer to Appendix A: The Formula Meal Plan Selection Chart.

50

AVOID
HIGH-CARBOHYDRATE
AIRLINE BREAKFASTS

If you often travel in airplanes, you're aware of the high-carbohydrate breakfast served by the airlines. The main reason for high-carbohydrate foods is obvious: they are much less expensive. Muffins, bagels, bananas, juice, sugary yogurt, and cereal are substantially less expensive to serve than a hot breakfast of bacon and eggs.

On one recent flight, we were served the breakfast that appears in the box on the next page.

With nothing better to do for the next several hours, we broke down the percentage of calories in this meal. As you can see, the meal contained a whopping 719 calories, of which 69% were from carbohydrate, 7% from protein, and 24% from fat. The majority of our fellow passengers ate all of the meal served and were fast asleep 30 to 40 minutes later. Maybe it's really part of a "How to get passengers to sleep during flights" conspiracy.

We try to avoid the high-carbohydrate breakfast food served on airplanes whenever possible and either eat before the flight, pack an egg burrito, or rely on a 40-30-30 Nutrition Bar. You can also bring hard-boiled eggs, Canadian bacon, or lowfat cottage cheese with you and eat only a portion of the high-carbohydrate breakfast served.

TYPICAL AIRLINE BREAKFAST

	Calories	Carbohydrates (grams)	Protein (grams)	Fat (grams)
6 ounces orange juice	88	22	0	0
1 banana	113	26	1	.5
Blueberry muffin	336	43	5	16
Fruit yogurt	182	33	7	2.5
Total grams		124	13	19
Calories per gram		x 4	x 4	x 9
Total calories	719	496	52	171
Percent of total calories		69%	7%	24%

The next time you have an early morning flight, plan ahead and make Gene's favorite Bacon and Egg Breakfast Burrito recipe on the following page. It's a delicious, balanced meal that will keep you awake and ready to take on the day.

Breakfast

	MEAL PLAN PERSONAL REQUIREMENTS*				
	A	B	C	D	E

KIDS' FAVORITE

Bacon and Egg Breakfast Burrito

	A	B	C	D	E
Egg, whole	1	1	1	1	1
Egg whites only	-	-	1	2	3
Canadian bacon	1 oz.	1 oz.	2 oz.	3 oz.	4½ oz.
Flour tortilla, 6- to 7-inch diameter	1	1	2	2½	3
Sour cream, lowfat	1 tbsp.	1 tbsp.	1½ tbsp.	2 tbsp.	3 tbsp.
Salsa	2 tbsp.	2 tbsp.	2 tbsp.	3 tbsp.	3 tbsp.

DIRECTIONS: Scramble eggs and whites in a nonstick pan. Cut Canadian bacon into strips and heat. Place cooked eggs, bacon, sour cream, and salsa in tortilla. Fold burrito-style and wrap tightly in plastic wrap. Delicious hot or cold.

For more than 200 personalized meals and recipes, including the Formula 40-30-30 Fat Flush Meals, refer to our book *The Formula*.

*To know your A, B, C, D, or E Meal Plan Personal Requirements, refer to Appendix A: The Formula Meal Plan Selection Chart.

51

INCLUDE LOWFAT COTTAGE CHEESE IN YOUR DIET

An excellent source of protein to include in your diet is cottage cheese. However, it does seem that cottage cheese is one of those foods that people either love or hate. We encourage those who love it to eat it often, and for those who don't like it, try to learn to like it. Why? Because lowfat cottage is truly a superfood that can make meal planning easier and can help make your body healthier and more fit.

Lowfat cottage cheese is a nutrient-dense powerhouse food. It is a good source of calcium and contains almost 40% of the RDA of Vitamin B-12. But what makes cottage cheese a superfood is that it is simply one of the best food sources of protein available. A half cup of cottage cheese supplies almost 15 grams of easy-to-digest, high-quality protein. It is also an easy protein food to chew, making it an excellent protein source for seniors. Lowfat cottage cheese is one of the richest sources of the amino acid lysine, which plays a critical role in supporting the immune system. Lysine is typically very low in vegetarian diets, making cottage cheese an excellent food for vegetarians. Lowfat cottage cheese supplies some of the highest amounts of the BCAAs (branch chain amino acids) of any food. BCAAs play a critical role in maintaining and building muscle. The more muscle you have, the higher your metabolism is and the more fat you burn, even while you sleep.

Lowfat cottage cheese is a convenient and economical source of protein. It requires no cooking, and can be eaten alone or mixed into many recipes. When compared to the price of other protein foods, cottage cheese is quite inexpensive.

On the following page is one of our favorite snacks. We love this snack when we are traveling. We refer to it as a "fast fruit meal" and think of it as an ultimate fast-food meal. You can buy the ingredients at any grocery store. Try this fast and easy recipe the next time you are in a hurry to put together a healthy balanced snack. This super fast-food meal also gives you the added benefit of being a Formula 40-30-30 Fat Flush meal, which can help you burn fat even faster.

Consider adding lowfat cottage cheese to your diet. It is a true superfood.

FORMULA 40-30-30 FAT FLUSH
MEAL PLAN PERSONAL REQUIREMENTS*

Snack

Lowfat Cottage Cheese with Fruit

	A	B	C	D	E
Knudsen on the Go! Lowfat 2% Milkfat Cottage Cheese (4-ounce cup)	1	1	1	1	2
Nuts (almonds, pecans, or walnuts)	2 tsp.	2 tsp.	2 tsp.	2 tsp.	1⅓ tbsp.
Apple, medium	½	½	½	½	1

DIRECTIONS: Mix together cottage cheese, nuts, and sliced apple.

For more than 200 personalized meals and recipes, including the Formula 40-30-30 Fat Flush Meals, refer to our book *The Formula*.

*To know your A, B, C, D, or E Meal Plan Personal Requirements, refer to Appendix A: The Formula Meal Plan Selection Chart.

52

REWARD YOURSELF

As your body fat decreases and muscle tone improves, we encourage you to set goals and plan personal reward days as you reach your goals. Actually write down your goals and make sure they are attainable.

Let's say that you've been following the Formula for two weeks and you've lost 10 pounds. Reward yourself by taking time to enjoy something special. Personal rewards can be as simple as a one-hour bubble bath with a scented candle and the door locked, or a massage at your favorite day spa. Choose little luxuries you don't normally indulge in so they are special ways of saying you're doing a great job. When you reach your goal and enjoy your reward, set a new goal. While you follow the Formula for the next few weeks, you can plan your next special reward.

Carol, one of our clients from Washington, told us that her husband began to treat her to personal reward days because he was so impressed with her success. As she continued to lose weight, he bought her a health club membership, a shopping spree, a day of beauty at the spa, and a tennis bracelet. When she reached her ideal weight, Carol didn't want her rewards to stop. She and her husband now enjoy tennis, running, biking, and hiking together. She says her favorite rewards aren't the gifts, but her revitalized relationship with her husband.

Your rewards don't have to be extravagant. They can be anything you enjoy. Listed below are several ideas to get you started:

- Bubble bath with no interruptions
- Manicure and pedicure
- Massage
- Body treatment: salt glow rub or mud bath
- Sauna or steam bath
- Foot massage
- Facial, at home or the spa
- A new outfit
- A sexy nightie
- Yoga classes
- A weekend getaway
- A hike in the woods
- A new pair of shoes
- A day of golf
- A hot air balloon ride
- Curling up with a good book or magazine

Start setting goals, achieving them, and rewarding yourself. It's a great way to stay motivated.

53

CHOOSE PRIMARILY FRUITS AND VEGETABLES FOR YOUR CARBOHYDRATE SOURCES

When you eat out or prepare your own meals, choose primarily fruits and vegetables (not starchy foods) for your carbohydrate sources. Fruits and vegetables are your best choice of carbohydrates for losing weight and burning fat.

The Formula uses the revolutionary 40-30-30 nutrition ratio: 40% of your total calories come from carbohydrates, 30% from protein, and 30% from fat. Since 1990, this nutrition ratio has helped millions of people from all walks of life to feel better and lose unwanted body fat. But just as important as the 40-30-30 ratio are the types of carbohydrates you choose.

Fruits and vegetables are loaded with healthy nutrients and contain only small amounts of carbohydrates, so it is very hard to overeat fruits and vegetables. For example, one cup of green beans contains about 10 grams of carbohydrates, while one average size potato contains 50 grams of carbohydrates. Even worse, the potato is a very high-glycemic food. Green beans, on the other hand, are a low-glycemic food. Most fruits and vegetables are low-glycemic because they contain fiber and their source of sugar is primarily fructose. Fructose increases blood sugar much more slowly than sucrose, the sugar that is found in starches. A potato will increase blood sugar 300% to 400% faster than green beans. Another way to look at it is that you can eat three to four times as many fruits and vegetables compared to starchy carbohydrates and still keep blood sugar balanced and burn fat.

Try the delicious recipe on the following page. It's a great source of low- to medium-glycemic fruits and vegetables and a Formula 40-30-30 Fat Flush dinner recipe.

FORMULA 40-30-30 FAT FLUSH
MEAL PLAN PERSONAL REQUIREMENTS*

Dinner

Citrus Spinach Salad

	A	B	C	D	E
Cooked chicken breast, cubed	3½ oz.	4 oz.	5 oz.	5 oz.	6 oz.
Baby spinach leaves, washed and dried	2½ cups	2½ cups	3 cups	3 cups	4 cups
Grapefruit, sections only	¾ cup	¾ cup	1 cup	1 cup	1¼ cups
Navel orange, peeled and sectioned	½ cup	¾ cup	¾ cup	¾ cup	1 cup
Avocado, medium, peeled and diced	3 tbsp.	3 tbsp.	¼ cup	¼ cup	⅓ cup

TANGERINE SHALLOT DRESSING RECIPE:

1 clove garlic

¼ teaspoon salt

2 tablespoons tangerine juice

2 tablespoons fresh lemon juice

1 tablespoon shallots, minced

½ tablespoon olive oil

RECIPE DIRECTIONS: Mash garlic with salt to make a paste. Place in a small jar and add tangerine and lemon juices, shallots, and olive oil and shake well. (Dressing recipe can be doubled or more, then split evenly if you make more than one portion of salad.)

DIRECTIONS: In a large bowl combine chicken, spinach leaves, grapefruit, and orange. Toss with Tangerine Shallot Dressing and serve topped with diced avocado.

For more than 200 personalized meals and recipes, including the Formula 40-30-30 Fat Flush Meals, refer to our book *The Formula*.

*To know your A, B, C, D, or E Meal Plan Personal Requirements, refer to Appendix A: The Formula Meal Plan Selection Chart.

54

NEVER, *EVER* GO INTO KETOSIS

Low-carbohydrate, high-protein diets promote what is called ketosis. You might lose some weight on diets that promote ketosis, but we have seen that much of the initial weight lost is water and muscle weight, with very little fat loss. To maximize fat burning and to lose the right kind of weight (fat, not muscle), it is best to avoid ketosis.

Ketosis is a metabolic process that occurs from not eating enough carbohydrates. The main reason to avoid ketosis is right between your ears: your brain! The main fuel for your brain and central nervous system is glucose. Glucose comes primarily from carbohydrate foods. When the body's limited carbohydrate stores are depleted, your brain starts to run out of fuel and protein is broken down to supply additional glucose. This protein comes from your diet or from lean body tissue such as organs and muscle. As the body attempts to conserve body proteins, it produces an alternative fuel source from the partial burning of fatty acids known as ketosis.

Ketone bodies are actually waste products (gases) from *incomplete fat* metabolism and serve as a glucose substitute for fueling the brain and central nervous system. As ketones break down, they accumulate in the blood and urine. These toxic waste products can make blood more acidic. The pH of the blood declines, upsetting the body's chemical balance, and excess ketone bodies can spill into the urine. This can cause unpleasant side effects such as headaches, dizziness, fatigue, low blood sugar, muscle wasting, and nausea. The body attempts to get rid of ketone bodies through increased urination, so much of the actual weight loss can be water loss and can lead to constipation. The water loss also leaches valuable electrolytes, like potassium, from the bloodstream and can contribute to leg cramps and muscle fatigue.

Even though you might burn some fat, ketosis can also turn your fat cells into fat magnets. This can cause you to easily regain any weight you might have lost as soon as you start eating carbohydrates again. In the early 1980s, after following a high-protein diet for six weeks for a bodybuilding contest, Gene gained more than 12 pounds in one night after he started to eat carbohydrates again. Not only was the six weeks of low carbohydrates and ketosis miserable, he lost lean muscle mass, his muscles looked flat, and he quickly regained all of the weight he had lost.

When you are in ketosis, you can break down valuable muscle protein simply to provide some glucose for your brain. Maintaining lean muscle mass is the key to an efficient metabolism, improving your ability to burn fat. Because you never, *ever* want to lose any amount of muscle, even a small amount, it makes absolutely no sense at all to follow a ketogenic diet.

Worst of all, ketosis stinks! As ketone gases start to ooze out of your body through your lungs and urine, it results in horrible body odor, bad breath, and a nasty taste in your mouth. We once spent three miserable hours on a plane next to man who was in ketosis. It is a foul smell you can't help but notice. We find it interesting that the promoters of ketogenic diets recommend using breath mints or gum to mask the foul, nasty smell.

We have worked with thousands of people who have followed high-protein diets and failed. Fortunately, most people simply cannot maintain such a restrictive diet for very long. To lose weight and to maximize fat burning, simply keep your diet balanced and avoid ketosis.

5 5

TRY A 40-30-30 NUTRITION BAR

One of the great breakthroughs in nutrition and food technology has been the introduction of 40-30-30 Nutrition Bars. Before 40-30-30 Nutrition Bars evolved, nutrition bars and diet bars were far too high in carbohydrates. But now you can buy a nutrition bar that is much more balanced. So, rather than having a high-carbohydrate bar or skipping meals and risking a drop in blood sugar, you can eat a 40-30-30 Nutrition Bar to help keep you balanced until your next meal.

40-30-30 Nutrition Bars derive 40% of their calories from carbohydrates, 30% from protein, and 30% from fat. They usually contain approximately 200 calories per bar and are fortified with vitamins and minerals. The balanced 40-30-30 nutrition ratio provides energy and helps keep your blood sugar balanced. The 30% high-quality protein helps turn on your fat-burning hormone glucagon, so you can burn fat faster. These bars are convenient when you simply do not have the time to prepare a balanced meal.

We were first introduced to 40-30-30 Nutrition Bars in 1991, when we were working with Dr. Barry Sears, the inventor of the world's first 40-30-30 Nutrition Bar. We began developing and testing the 40-30-30 nutrition program at our clinic, the BioSyn Human Performance Center, located in Kirkland, Washington. We were simply amazed at how well the original "Tootsie Roll®" size bars worked for us. We were both very active professionals. We had just recently changed our diets to the 40-30-30 zone ratio and were experiencing great results, but when we started using the Nutrition Bars, it made following the program even easier. We continued to lose body fat and gain muscle mass, had more energy, and felt better. We still use 40-30-30 Nutrition Bars daily and wouldn't think of traveling without them.

Listed below is an approximate nutritional profile for a 40-30-30 Nutrition Bar. Use this sample when shopping for a balanced nutrition bar:

40-30-30 Nutrition Bar Nutritional Profile

190–200 calories

20 grams carbohydrate (40% of total calories)

14 grams protein (30% of total calories)

6 grams fat (30% of total calories)

There are several companies that make 40-30-30 Nutrition Bars. The bars that we use and recommend are the Balance Bar by the Balance Bar Company, The Ironman Triathlon Bar by Twin Laboratories, Inc., the PR Bar by PR Nutrition Inc., and the 40-30-30 Bar by Trader Joe's. These bars come in many flavors and are available at most health food stores, grocery stores, drug stores, and convenience stores.

40-30-30 Nutrition Bars make following the Formula so easy anyone can do it. The next time you are in a rush, don't skip meals—instead, eat a 40-30-30 Nutrition Bar.

56

KEEP IT SIMPLE

Many people try to make following the Formula difficult. Our mantra is, "Keep It Simple." When you begin following the Formula, don't get confused by spending a lot of time counting food blocks or calculating carbohydrate, protein, and fat grams when preparing 40-30-30 meals. Rather, use the meals we have prepared and personalized for you. There are many new recipes in this book and hundreds of recipes in *The Formula* to choose from. Each has been broken down into the appropriate serving size for you and other family members.

Begin by choosing one or two meals you like from the breakfast, lunch, snack, and dinner categories and make them often. Once you have mastered making your favorite few meals, you can begin to introduce a wider variety of meals or begin to design your own. Just remember: the Formula is easy to follow when you keep it simple.

Try this delicious new Family Style pizza dinner recipe using a Boboli Thin Crust Pizza Crust. It's quick and easy to prepare and is simply delicious. Enjoy it with a salad.

MEAL PLAN PERSONAL REQUIREMENTS*

Dinner
Family Style
Big Ruma's Garlic Chicken Pizza

	A	B	C	D	E
Big Ruma's Garlic Chicken Pizza (recipe below)	2 slices	2½ slices	3 slices	3 slices	4 slices
Mixed salad greens	2 cups	2 cups	2 cups	2 cups	2 cups
Cherry tomatoes	5	5	5	5	5
Italian salad dressing	1 tbsp.	1 tbsp.	1 tbsp.	1 tbsp.	1 tbsp.

BIG RUMA'S GARLIC CHICKEN PIZZA RECIPE:

1 Boboli Thin Pizza Crust, 10-ounce
2½ cups diced cooked chicken breast
1 large jalapeño pepper, diced
3 cloves garlic, diced
¼ cup diced green onion
¼ cup diced red onion
½ cup chopped fresh basil
½ cup chopped fresh cilantro
2 tablespoons Parmesan cheese
1 tablespoon olive oil

RECIPE DIRECTIONS: Preheat oven to 450°F. Place crust on an ungreased cookie sheet. In a large bowl, add diced chicken, jalapeño pepper, garlic, onion, basil, and cilantro. Toss to blend. Pour on top of Boboli Crust and spread evenly. Sprinkle with Parmesan cheese and olive oil. Bake 10–12 minutes. Cut into 8 even slices to serve.

DIRECTIONS: Serve pizza with salad, tomatoes and dressing. *Note:* This recipe was designed by Joyce's brother, John Buhmann. We named it for him. Thanks, John.

For more than 200 personalized meals and recipes, including the Formula 40-30-30 Fat Flush Meals, refer to our book *The Formula*.

*To know your A, B, C, D, or E Meal Plan Personal Requirements, refer to Appendix A: The Formula Meal Plan Selection Chart.

57

PARK AT THE BACK
OF PARKING LOTS

For an easy way to get some extra exercise (for some people, this might be their only exercise), try parking at the back of parking lots. Gene has been doing it for years.

We all know that exercise is good for you, but some people find it hard to find the time to incorporate exercise in their busy lifestyle. So, instead of parking up close in parking lots, park as far away as possible, as often as possible, and use this opportunity to exercise. Walk briskly and with purpose, and you will be amazed at how easy it is to get in some extra exercise. You will also get the added benefit of not getting your car all dinged up from people parking next to you.

Instead of using the escalator or elevator, take the stairs whenever possible. Think of these situations as an opportunity to easily and almost effortlessly increase your activity. In no time at all, it will become a new, heart-healthy habit.

Walking can be a perfect time to practice affirmations that help you focus on your goals. Gene uses *fit, lean, fat-burning machine*. Repeat your affirmation to yourself as you walk, and you will be getting the added bene-fit of positive thinking and "the mind-muscle link."

So forget trying to find a close parking spot and start parking at the back of the parking lot. It's not only good for your health, it's good for your car.

58

LEARN HOW TO MAKE YOUR FAVORITE RESTAURANT SALADS

Have you ever eaten a delicious specialty salad in a restaurant and wished you could duplicate it at home? We do it almost every time we eat out. In fact, Joyce is great at ordering meals that are already close to 40-30-30. If they aren't, you can leave out some carbohydrates or add some to make it Formula perfect.

You can find delicious specialty salads in restaurants that offer Mexican and Southwest cuisine. When you find one that you want to make at home, jot down the ingredients. We even ask what the dressing was made from so duplicating it is easier. Unless it's their "secret sauce," restaurants are usually glad to tell you. If the salad is served on a large tortilla or in a deep-fried tortilla shell, you can make substitutions that conform to the Formula principles. Many restaurant specialty salads are served in huge portions. Adjust your home version to meet your Formula personal requirements.

Enjoy one of Joyce's favorite finds: Chipotle Chicken Salad. It's delicious for lunch or dinner.

MEAL PLAN PERSONAL REQUIREMENTS*

Lunch or Dinner

Chipotle Chicken Salad

	A	B	C	D	E
Romaine lettuce, cleaned and torn	6 leaves	6 leaves	8 leaves	8 leaves	8 leaves
Cooked chicken breast, cut into strips	¾ cup	1 cup	1 cup	1 cup	1⅓ cups
Corn, canned or fresh (cooked)	¼ cup	¼ cup	¼ cup	¼ cup	⅓ cup
Black beans, canned, drained	¼ cup	¼ cup	¼ cup	¼ cup	⅓ cup
Jicama, peeled and chopped	¼ cup	¼ cup	¼ cup	¼ cup	¼ cup
Apple, diced	⅓ cup	½ cup	½ cup	½ cup	½ cup
Tomato, diced	¼ cup	¼ cup	½ cup	½ cup	½ cup
Chipotle Salad Dressing (recipe below)	2½ tbsp.	2½ tbsp.	2½ tbsp.	2½ tbsp.	3 tbsp.
Tortilla, baked strips, 7-inch diameter	½ tortilla	½ tortilla	⅔ tortilla	⅔ tortilla	1 tortilla

CHIPOTLE SALAD DRESSING RECIPE:

2 tablespoons Chipotle peppers in Adobo sauce, canned

2 tablespoons olive oil

1 tablespoon red wine vinegar

2 tablespoons orange juice

1 teaspoon fresh lime juice

Salt and pepper to taste

RECIPE DIRECTIONS: In a food processor or blender, process all ingredients until creamy.

DIRECTIONS: Cut tortilla into confetti-style strips and bake until crisp in a 350° oven. In a large salad bowl, place lettuce, chicken, corn, beans, Jicama, apple, and tomato and toss with Chipotle Salad Dressing. Transfer to a serving plate and top with baked tortilla strips.

For more than 200 personalized meals and recipes, including the Formula 40-30-30 Fat Flush Meals, refer to our book *The Formula*.

*To know your A, B, C, D, or E Meal Plan Personal Requirements, refer to Appendix A: The Formula Meal Plan Selection Chart.

59

DON'T WEIGH YOURSELF SO OFTEN

There are several ways to track your results when following the Formula. The most misleading is jumping on a bathroom scale. A scale can tell you only your overall body weight. But there is a big difference between losing weight and losing fat. If your goal is to lose weight, you actually want to lose fat without the loss of muscle mass. You never want to lose muscle or sacrifice other body proteins in an attempt to simply lose weight. You always want to lose fat. So forget the scale and use an alternative method.

The most accurate method to track fat loss is to have your body fat tested. There are many types of machines that test body fat. Use the system you like best. Healthy and fit men should test around 15% body fat or less, and women should be around 20% body fat or less. The men we tested averaged more than 25% and women were more than 35%. Have your body fat tested about every 30 days. When Gene began following the Formula, he lost 12 pounds of pure fat and gained 5 pounds of solid muscle. Even though the scale only went down by 7 pounds, his results were simply awesome! Have you ever seen what 12 pounds of fat looks like? It's huge! You will not believe how great you look and feel when you lose 12 pounds of pure fat, regardless of what the scale says.

Another method to use is what we call "The Naked Mirror Test." Once a week, simply get naked and check out your body in front of a full-length mirror. Be honest with yourself and review your body for any improvements.

Another simple method is what we call "The Tight Jeans Test." Once a week, try on a pair of your tightest-fitting jeans. Judge your results by how the jeans fit. As they become looser, you are losing fat.

If your body fat percentage is coming down, or if you are looking great standing naked in front of your mirror, or your tight jeans are fitting looser, you are losing body fat. Forget the bathroom scale. These alternative methods will be more accurate at monitoring your fat loss, while you keep your muscle.

60

LEARN WHAT BEVERAGES WORK BEST

The calories and carbohydrates found in many beverages play a critical role when it comes to losing weight and burning fat. To maximize your body's natural ability to burn stored body fat for energy, you should learn what beverages to drink.

Soft drinks, bottled teas, juices, sports drinks, and the like are typically very high in carbohydrates. These drinks are a major source of empty calories. Their overconsumption is considered a major cause of the rapid rise of obesity and diabetes in this country, especially in children.

Plainly stated, high-carbohydrate, sugary beverages can get you fat and keep you fat. Too many carbohydrates spike blood sugar and stimulate the hormone insulin. Excess insulin converts excess glucose into stored body fat. So, if your goal is to lose weight and burn fat, minimize the high-carbohydrate beverages you drink.

Many athletes rely on high-carbohydrate sports drinks to increase electrolyte consumption. They can also help prevent muscle cramps. If you can't give up sports drinks, reduce their carbohydrates dramatically by diluting the drink with one-half to two-thirds as much water. When Gene is training for a competition, he uses sports drinks during his training, but dilutes them with plenty of water.

Pure water, of course, is the very best beverage to drink. In fact, try drinking nothing but pure water for two weeks. Feel free to spice it up with a wedge of lemon or lime. You will be amazed at how good you feel and at the improvement in your skin. But many people like to have more options than just water. With that in mind, listed below are suitable beverages to drink when following the Formula.

Beverages That Work Best When Following the Formula:

- Pure water
- Mineral water
- Seltzer or club soda
- Milk, lowfat or nonfat
- Decaffeinated tea (hot or cold)
- Decaffeinated coffee (hot or cold)
- Iced lowfat decaffeinated latte (excess caffeine can stimulate insulin)
- Sugar-free, caffeine-free soft drinks

61

LIMIT OR ELIMINATE CAFFEINE

The Formula is a balanced diet that can help stabilize blood sugar and begin to control insulin. Excess caffeine has been shown to elevate insulin. Caffeine is a central nervous system stimulant and a diuretic, and too much can be harmful.

Coffee, tea, many soft drinks, and chocolate all contain caffeine in varying amounts. Coffee has been the major dietary source of caffeine in the American diet since 1773. The amount of caffeine per serving varies with the variety of coffee bean used, the coffee grind, the method and length of brewing, and whether the coffee is regular or instant. Dark roasted coffee, like the kind you buy in gourmet coffee shops, actually contains less caffeine than the lighter roasts. Tea leaves contain a higher concentration of caffeine than coffee by weight, but less tea is required to make a cup. The longer tea is brewed, the higher the caffeine content. Herbal teas provide a caffeine-free alternative to coffee and tea. They are primarily brewed from flowers, leaves, seeds, or the bark or roots of plants and can include lemon, orange, or apple and spices like cinnamon, ginger, and mint.

Soft drinks are the number-one source of added sugar in the American diet and are the second greatest source of caffeine. Many children consume more caffeine from soft drinks per body weight than adults do from coffee. If you have been consuming large amounts of caffeine from coffee, tea, or colas throughout the day, begin to cut back gradually. To avoid caffeine withdrawal headaches, make a blend of half regular and half decaffeinated coffee. Look for organic beans that have been decaffeinated by using a water process. After a few weeks, use only 25% regular coffee. Eventually, you will be drinking only decaffeinated. Colas also come decaffeinated and, depending on the volume consumed, should be switched slowly as well.

Another way to control the insulin-elevating effects of caffeine is to drink your beverage with a balanced meal.

62

LEARN HOW TO MAKE 40-30-30 COFFEE DRINKS

It's rather obvious that Americans love coffee drinks. Cappuccinos, mochas, lattes, either hot or iced, are so popular, many people make them a daily habit. Unfortunately, many of them can be loaded with sugar. This added source of high-carbohydrate calories can spike blood sugar levels and get you out of your fat-burning zone.

Also, too much caffeine can spike insulin, so use caffeine in moderation or use decaf.

We are asked how to make coffee drinks work with the Formula so often that we began to experiment and came up with several solutions. One recommendation is to have a small drink and enjoy it with half of a 40-30-30 Nutrition Bar as a balanced afternoon snack.

If you love coffee drinks, try some of the 40-30-30 Formula blends we've come up with.

Joyce's favorite is a hot or iced latte from Starbucks. A latte contains steamed milk with a shot of espresso. Lowfat milk is naturally close to the 40-30-30 ratio. To turn the latte into a chocolate mocha, sprinkle with cocoa powder and add half a packet of a low-calorie sweetener.

A SHORT, DECAFFEINATED, NONFAT LATTE

	Calories	Carbohydrates	Protein	Fat
6 ounces steamed milk, 2% lowfat	100	10	7	3.5
1 shot of decaffeinated espresso	0	0	0	0
Total in grams		10	7	3.5
		x 4	x 4	x 9
Total calories	100	40	28	31.5
Percentage of calories		40%	28%	31.5%

At home, try these recipes.

40-30-30 HOT MOCHA

	Calories	Carbohydrates	Protein	Fat
3 tablespoons Nescafé Frothé Chocolate Mocha Mix	82	14	1	2.5
10 grams pure whey protein powder	40	0	10	0
1 teaspoon whipped cream	18	0	0	2
Total in grams		14	11	4.5
		x 4	x 4	x 9
Total calories	140	56	44	40.5
Percentage of calories		40%	31%	29%

DIRECTIONS: Place 3 level tablespoons of mocha mix in a cup with 10 grams of whey protein powder. Stir dry ingredients to blend. While stirring, add 8 ounces of boiling water until blended. Top with whipped cream. *Note:* For more information on pure whey protein, please refer to the Appendix at the back of the book.

40-30-30 ICED MOCHA

	Calories	Carbohydrates	Protein	Fat
4.75 ounces Starbucks Frappuccino Mocha, lowfat (half a bottle)	100	17.5	3.5	1.75
10 grams pure whey protein powder	40	0	10	0
¾ cup crushed ice	0	0	0	0
2 teaspoons Macadamia nuts, chopped	39	.5	.25	4
Total in grams		18	13.75	5.75
		x 4	x 4	x 9
Total Calories	179	72	55	51.75
Percentage of calories		40%	31%	29%

DIRECTIONS: Combine all ingredients in a blender and process until smooth. *Note:* For more information on pure whey protein, please refer to Appendix C: Special Ingredients.

The above coffee drinks are suitable as a midafternoon snack with half of a 40-30-30 Nutrition Bar.

63

CONSIDER BEANS AND RICE AS A CARBOHYDRATE SOURCE

Many people think of the combination of beans and rice as a high-protein food. Beans and rice each contain a small amount of incomplete protein that can be combined to obtain a complete protein, but these foods are predominantly carbohydrates.

A half cup of black beans contains approximately 20 grams of carbohydrate, 8 grams of protein, and <1 gram of fat. More than 70% of the total calories are from carbohydrates. Rice is even higher. A half cup of rice contains approximately 26 grams of carbohydrate, 3 grams of protein, and <1 gram of fat. More than 89% of the total calories are from carbohydrates. When you combine the two, they contain approximately 80% of the total calories from carbohydrates.

Beans and rice are healthy foods that can be included in any balanced diet, but they should be considered a source of carbohydrate, not protein. Use them in conjunction with low-fat, high-quality protein and good fat. Because beans and rice are both high-starch carbohydrates, we recommend using only one in a meal along with lower glycemic carbohydrates.

Enjoy Beef Kabobs with Fried Rice for a delicious, perfect balance of carbohydrates, protein, and fat.

Dinner

KIDS' FAVORITE

Beef Kabobs with Fried Rice

	MEAL PLAN PERSONAL REQUIREMENTS*				
	A	B	C	D	E
Top loin beef, extra-lean, cubed	3 oz.	3½ oz.	4½ oz.	4½ oz.	5½ oz.
Teriyaki marinade, bottled	1 tbsp.	1 tbsp.	2 tbsp.	2 tbsp.	2 tbsp.
Fried Rice (see below)					
Green or red bell pepper, medium, cubed	⅓	⅓	½	½	½
Sweet onion, cubed	¼	¼	½	½	½
Cherry tomatoes	4	4	6	6	6

FRIED RICE RECIPE:

	A	B	C	D	E
Brown and wild rice blend, uncooked	3 tbsp.	¼ cup	¼ cup	¼ cup	⅓ cup
Beef broth, canned	½ cup	½ cup	½ cup	½ cup	⅔ cup
Olive oil	1½ tsp.	1½ tsp.	2 tsp.	2 tsp.	2 tsp.
Carrots, diced	2 tbsp.	3 tbsp.	¼ cup	¼ cup	¼ cup
Celery, diced	2 tbsp.	3 tbsp.	¼ cup	¼ cup	¼ cup

RECIPE DIRECTIONS: Cook rice in beef broth. In a frying pan, heat oil and sauté carrots and celery until tender. Add cooked rice and toss to blend.

DIRECTIONS: Marinate beef cubes in teriyaki marinade for 20–30 minutes. On several skewers, alternate marinated beef cubes, bell pepper, onion, and tomatoes. Grill or broil and serve with fried rice.

For more than 200 personalized meals and recipes, including the Formula 40-30-30 Fat Flush Meals, refer to our book *The Formula*.

*To know your A, B, C, D, or E Meal Plan Personal Requirements, refer to Appendix A: The Formula Meal Plan Selection Chart.

64

CONSIDER NUTS AND SEEDS AS A FAT SOURCE

Many people, especially vegetarians, consider nuts and seeds as high-protein foods. Nuts and seeds contain small amounts of protein and small amounts of carbohydrates, but are highest in fat. They should be classified as fat, not protein.

One ounce of most nuts or seeds contains about 15 to 20 grams of high-quality fat and only about 3 to 6 grams of protein. Approximately 70% to 80% of the total calories in nuts and seeds are from fat. Because they are so high in fat, they should be used in small amounts in meals and recipes.

Nuts and seeds are included in many of our recipes. They give the recipe a great flavor. The fat they contain triggers a hormonal response that helps keep you full, keeps blood sugar balanced, and supplies important essential fatty acids for proper hormone production.

The Yogurt Blend recipe on the following page is a delicious breakfast that includes nuts. It is fast and easy to prepare, as well as light and nutritious. Yogurt and cottage cheese create a high-quality, easy-to-digest protein. The fruit is a low-glycemic carbohydrate food and the nuts are a high-quality fat. As you can see, it's easy to add a small amount of nuts to a meal to make it balanced and healthy.

Breakfast

KIDS' FAVORITE

Yogurt Blend

	FORMULA 40-30-30 FAT FLUSH MEAL PLAN PERSONAL REQUIREMENTS*				
	A	B	C	D	E
Yogurt (Knudsen Cal 70), any flavor	1 cup	1 cup	1 cup	1 cup	1 cup
Cottage cheese, 2% lowfat	¼ cup	¼ cup	⅓ cup	⅔ cup	¾ cup
Apple, medium, sliced	⅓	⅓	½	1	1
Nuts (almonds, pecans, or walnuts)	1⅓ tbsp.	1⅓ tbsp.	2 tbsp.	2½ tbsp.	3 tbsp.

DIRECTIONS: Combine fruit-flavored yogurt with cottage cheese and apple. Sprinkle with nuts.

For more than 200 personalized meals and recipes, including the Formula 40-30-30 Fat Flush Meals, refer to our book *The Formula*.

*To know your A, B, C, D, or E Meal Plan Personal Requirements, refer to Appendix A: The Formula Meal Plan Selection Chart.

65

HAVE A
FLASHBACK DAY

After they have been following the Formula plan for several months, we encourage clients to review their original journal pages. We call it a Flashback Day.

Review the first day of your journal, specifically any notes you made on how you felt at that time, such as energy levels, sleep patterns, and moods. It's also a good time to retest your body fat and take measurements. If you are monitoring blood pressure and cholesterol, see your doctor for a new blood panel and jot down your improvements. Notice if you are feeling better, thinking more clearly, or if your memory has improved.

If you are a woman, do your hormones seem more balanced and have moods improved? Have any PMS symptoms improved or disappeared, such as bloating, water retention, moodiness, sugar cravings, cramps, and headaches? Do your clothes fit better? Are your love handles gone? Are you more active? Has stamina improved? Do you feel well-rested on less sleep? Do you wake up more easily and no longer get sleepy in the afternoon?

If you're experiencing any or all of these benefits, you are realizing the power of food and the Formula. When you flash back to the way you used to feel, you realize how good a balanced diet makes you feel. Flashback Days are a great way to boost your motivation to follow the Formula for a lifetime.

66

WHEN YOU EAT OUT, CHOOSE WISELY

◆

Statistics show that Americans eat out an average of 30% of the time. Studies show that people who dine out often have more body fat than people who eat at home. With 38% of Americans overweight, that's 106.9 million people increasing their risk for diabetes, obesity, heart disease, arthritis, osteoporosis, high blood pressure, high cholesterol, and certain types of cancer.

One problem with eating out is the extra-large portions we are being served. They are high in carbohydrates and high in fat. It has also been reported that 67% of Americans eat everything on their plate.

When you decide to dine out on a supersize "value" meal, split it with a friend or eat only half and bring the rest home for a leftover meal the next day. Order your meal without bread, chips, or starchy vegetables. Choose a lowfat protein like grilled chicken or fish, a large salad with the dressing served on the side, and a large serving of steamed vegetables like broccoli, asparagus, green beans, or an artichoke. Drink water and a beverage such as iced tea with lemon or sparkling bottled water with lime. If you want an alcoholic beverage, one glass of red or white wine or a light beer are your best choices. Also, drink it with your meal rather than before.

When eating in a fast-food restaurant, choose your meal wisely. A grilled chicken sandwich is a much better choice than a hamburger. Avoid the fries and onion rings. Wendy's chili is an almost perfect 40-30-30 Formula meal and one of Joyce's favorites. Grilled fish tacos are Gene's favorite. Sandwich shops also make a fairly balanced turkey sandwich when you order double turkey.

When you eat out, you have choices to make. Choose your meal wisely and it's easy to follow the Formula.

67

HOW TO MAKE IT THROUGH THE HOLIDAYS

Did you know that 51% of the annual weight gain occurs during the six-week holiday season Thanksgiving to New Year's? The average weight gain during the holidays is at least 5 pounds, and most people don't lose it. There are 106.9 million Americans already classified as overweight or obese. Add 5 more pounds, holiday stress, and the lack of exercise, and the holidays for many can be quite dangerous. Maybe it's time to make some changes for yourself as well as your family and friends.

The trouble with overeating during the holidays is not just the added calories, but more specifically, the extra carbohydrates found in cookies, candies, fruitcakes, and holiday drinks. The added sugar load causes blood sugar and insulin levels to rise, promoting fat storage. In just a few weeks, your pants fit tighter and energy levels suffer. But it doesn't have to be that way.

When you attend holiday office parties, cocktail parties, or family gatherings, take the time to balance the foods you eat and drink. Begin by looking for the protein first. If you are going to drink a high-carbohydrate drink or an alcoholic beverage, eat protein appetizers with your drink. Fill your plate with protein foods like meatballs, chicken skewers, sliced turkey or ham, salmon, sushi, and cheese. Fresh fruit and raw vegetables are also good choices, as they contain very few carbohydrates. Avoid breads, crackers, chips, cookies, candy, and other rich desserts to keep your blood sugar balanced.

Remember this advice during the holidays and you will never have to worry about gaining those extra, energy-zapping 5 pounds. In fact, many of our clients have been amazed that they were able to continue losing weight during the holidays while still enjoying delicious foods.

68

BUY SLICED DELI MEATS IN PREMEASURED 4-OUNCE PACKS

When you buy a pound of sliced deli meat, ask the butcher to put a sheet of deli tissue between every 4 ounces. This way, when you are preparing a Formula meal that requires 4 ounces of deli meat, it is already premeasured for you. If you need only 2 ounces, it's easy to cut it in half, so you will know exactly how much meat you are using.

This method teaches you portion control. Four ounces of most lean meats contain approximately 0 carbohydrates, 25 grams of high-quality protein, and 2 grams of fat (for a 0-90-10 ratio). In very little time, you will become adept in portioning deli meat for your own personal requirements without needing a scale.

One of Gene's favorite snacks is the Tortilla Roll-up on the following page. He has been recommending it for years because it's fast, easy to prepare, and delicious.

Snack	MEAL PLAN PERSONAL REQUIREMENTS*				
	A	B	C	D	E

KIDS' FAVORITE

Tortilla Roll-Up

	A	B	C	D	E
Flour tortilla, 7- to 8-inch diameter	1	1	1	1	2
Mayonnaise, full-fat	1 tsp.	1 tsp.	1 tsp.	1 tsp.	2 tsp.
Lean deli meat (turkey, chicken, or roast beef)	2 ½ oz.	2 ½ oz.	2 ½ oz.	2 ½ oz.	5 oz.

DIRECTIONS: Spread flour tortilla with mayonnaise. Top with deli meat and roll it up.

For more than 200 personalized meals and recipes, including the Formula 40-30-30 Fat Flush Meals, refer to our book *The Formula.*

*To know your A, B, C, D, or E Meal Plan Personal Requirements, refer to Appendix A: The Formula Meal Plan Selection Chart.

69

TURN ANY MEAL INTO A FORMULA 40-30-30 FAT FLUSH MEAL

The Formula is based on two principles: individual requirements and balanced nutrition. Your sex, weight, and activity level determine the overall amount of food and number of calories you need daily to maximize the burning of stored fat for energy. The A, B, and C plans are typically used by women, the C, D, and E plans by men. Each personalized plan provides appropriate portions for your individual requirements.

The ratio of carbohydrate, protein, and fat calories in a meal helps control blood sugar stabilization from meal to meal and its resulting hormonal response. *The Formula* provides both Regular and Formula 40-30-30 Fat Flush meals. Both contain the 40-30-30 Formula ratio, but Regular meals include a greater variety of low-, medium-, and high-glycemic carbohydrates, while Formula 40-30-30 Fat Flush meals contain only low- to medium-glycemic carbohydrates. Formula 40-30-30 Fat Flush meals are a way to severely tighten the control of blood sugar levels and balance body chemistry to its highest fat-burning potential.

You can turn any Regular Meal into a Formula 40-30-30 Fat Flush meal simply by substituting the high-glycemic carbohydrates for lower-glycemic carbohydrates. If a Regular 40-30-30 breakfast includes eggs, toast, and fruit, you can turn it into a Formula 40-30-30 Fat Flush breakfast by replacing the toast with a low-glycemic carbohydrate such as a sliced tomato.

Breakfast Example

REGULAR MEAL, B-PLAN

1 whole egg

2 egg whites

1 tablespoon cheddar cheese, ⅓ less fat, shredded

1 slice whole wheat toast, reduced calorie

1 orange

FORMULA 40-30-30 FAT FLUSH MEAL, B-PLAN

1 whole egg

2 egg whites

1 tablespoon cheddar cheese, ⅓ less fat, shredded

1 sliced tomato, medium size

1 orange

Enjoy either a Regular meal or a Formula 40-30-30 Fat Flush meal using the Hawaiian Chicken Salad recipe on the following page.

FORMULA 40-30-30 FAT FLUSH

Lunch
Family Style
Hawaiian Chicken Salad with Fruit

MEAL PLAN PERSONAL REQUIREMENTS*	A	B	C	D	E
Hawaiian Chicken Salad (recipe below)	⅔ cup	1 cup	1 cup	1¼ cups	1½ cups
Red leaf lettuce, cleaned and dried	2 leaves	3 leaves	3 leaves	3 leaves	3 leaves
Papaya or strawberries	½ cup	¾ cup	¾ cup	¾ cup	½ cup
Kiwi, large, peeled	1	1	1	1	2

DIRECTIONS: Place Hawaiian Chicken Salad on lettuce leaves and serve with fresh sliced fruit.

Lunch
Hawaiian Chicken Salad Wraps

MEAL PLAN PERSONAL REQUIREMENTS*	A	B	C	D	E
Hawaiian Chicken Salad (recipe on following page)	½ cup	¾ cup	¾ cup	1 cup	1¼ cups
Red leaf lettuce, cleaned and dried	1 leaf	2 leaves	2 leaves	2 leaves	2 leaves
Whole wheat, lowfat tortilla, 6- or 9-inch (La Tortilla Factory)	1, 6-inch	2, 6-inch	2, 6-inch	1, 6-inch and 1, 9-inch	2, 9-inch
Grapes, red	¼ cup	½ cup	½ cup	½ cup	½ cup

DIRECTIONS: Place Hawaiian Chicken Salad and lettuce on whole wheat tortillas. Roll and serve with grapes.

HAWAIIAN CHICKEN SALAD RECIPE:

4 cups chicken breast, cooked and cubed

¾ cup diced celery

⅓ cup diced red onion

⅓ cup diced green onion

4 pineapple rings, chopped

¼ cup chopped macadamia nuts

¼ cup mayonnaise, lowfat

RECIPE DIRECTIONS: Add all ingredients in a bowl and toss to combine.

For more than 200 personalized meals and recipes, including the Formula 40-30-30 Fat Flush Meals, refer to our book *The Formula*.

*To know your A, B, C, D, or E Meal Plan Personal Requirements, refer to Appendix A: The Formula Meal Plan Selection Chart.

70

CHOOSING THE VERY BEST EXERCISE

What's the best exercise for shaping up and losing fat? That's simple: Whatever exercise you can enjoy and stick with. If you hate to run, chances are you won't do it. Choose any form of exercise that you enjoy, schedule your time, and stick with it. If you find yourself getting bored, try something new.

It's important to set realistic exercise goals. Exercise can instantly boost self-esteem and fitness levels. Vigorous exercise releases endorphins, brain chemicals that relieve pain and induce a mild sense of euphoria. You just feel better after exercise. But realistic goals are important. If you are a sedentary person and you achieve your goal of walking twice around the track, you are likely to feel an immediate sense of achievement and self-esteem. But, if you attempt to run two laps the first time out and fail, you may become frustrated and give up. When you set realistic exercise goals and reach them, you inevitably boost self-confidence. As exercise becomes routine, push yourself to reach new goals. Many people walk around in a state of unconscious tension. But exercise of any kind, by tensing muscles and then relaxing them, can become a powerful tool to reduce daily stress, fatigue, and tension. Exercise can help you shape up both physically and mentally.

Exercise and a balanced diet provide the perfect combination for lowering your risk of disease, improving heart health, reversing aging, and increasing self-esteem. Find the exercise you enjoy, set your exercise goals, and just do it.

71

INCLUDE BARLEY IN YOUR DIET

◆

When you think of starchy grains and vegetables, you typically think of potatoes, rice, and pasta. These are the high-glycemic carbohydrate foods that have been labeled "bad foods" by the high-protein dieters. We don't like to exclude any foods on the Formula, especially foods that have been thought of as staples in the American diet for years. Sweet potatoes and yams, wild and brown rice, and whole grain pasta are nutrient dense, fiber filled carbohydrate foods and should be part of a healthy, balanced diet.

But there's a new kid on the block that has gained a whole new respect in the low-glycemic world of grains: barley. Although barley is a carbohydrate-dense food (½ cup cooked barley contains 22 grams of carbohydrates), it is a rich source of soluble fiber to help reduce blood cholesterol levels and is low-glycemic.

We use cooked barley in place of potatoes or rice. It has a distinct roasted flavor and can easily be added to salads and soups or served as a side dish, plain or with a dash of soy sauce. Cook 1 cup of barley with 3 cups of water, vegetable broth, or chicken stock with ½ teaspoon salt.

Enjoy one of our favorite Family Style soup recipes that contains barley.

FORMULA 40-30-30 FAT FLUSH
MEAL PLAN PERSONAL REQUIREMENTS*

Dinner

KIDS' FAVORITE/ *Family Style*

Beef Barley Soup and Salad

	A	B	C	D	E
Beef Barley Soup (recipe below)	2 cups	2¼ cups	2⅔ cups	2⅔ cups	3⅓ cups
Mixed salad greens	2 cups	2½ cups	3 cups	3 cups	3 cups
Oil and vinegar salad dressing	1 tbsp.	1 tbsp.	1⅓ tbsp.	1⅓ tbsp.	1⅔ tbsp.

BEEF BARLEY SOUP RECIPE:

1½ pounds boneless beef chuck

5 cups water

3 cups canned beef broth

2 cups chopped mushroom pieces

2 cups chopped celery

1 cup chopped onion

1 cup chopped zucchini

1 teaspoon salt

½ teaspoon crushed dried rosemary

½ teaspoon pepper

1 clove garlic, minced

6 ounces tomato paste

1 cup pearl barley

RECIPE DIRECTIONS: Trim meat of all visible fat and cut into ¾-inch cubes. Combine all ingredients in a Dutch oven or large pot. Bring to a full boil, reduce heat, cover and simmer for 1½ hours. *Note:* You can subsitute chicken or turkey if you prefer.

DIRECTIONS: Measure appropriate portions of Beef Barley Soup using a measuring cup. Serve soup with salad and olive oil and vinegar dressing.

For more than 200 personalized meals and recipes, including the Formula 40-30-30 Fat Flush Meals, refer to our book *The Formula*.

*To know your A, B, C, D, or E Meal Plan Personal Requirements, refer to Appendix A: The Formula Meal Plan Selection Chart.

72

USE SEASONAL FRUITS AND VEGETABLES

When a recipe calls for a specific fruit or vegetable as part of the carbohydrates, you can always substitute equal amounts of a comparable fruit or vegetable. In fact, it's a good idea to choose fruits and vegetables from those that are in season. Prices will usually be lower and the food will be fresher.

Small, young vegetables and fruits often have more flavor and more nutrients per pound than do larger ones because nutrients are usually concentrated near the surface. The darker, more colorful produce generally has the highest nutrients. Fresh produce that sits in the refrigerator for too long can lose taste and nutrients.

We shop for seasonal produce several times per week. Spring is a great time to load up on strawberries and asparagus. Summer melons are delicious and easy to cut into chunks or balls and freeze. We buy blueberries, raspberries, blackberries, and peaches when they are in season and on sale, then freeze them for shakes and fruit salads. You can support your local farmers market for the freshest produce. That's where you can find tomatoes that actually taste like tomatoes. You can make your own tomato sauce and freeze or can it. Farmers markets in fall offer many varieties of fresh squash, peppers, and greens.

Apples, oranges, grapes, lettuce, broccoli, and other fruits and vegetables can be found pretty much year-round. But, whenever possible, choose organic fruits and vegetables, grown without the use of chemicals, fertilizers, and pesticides. Many grocery stores now provide organic produce sections. In many cases, it may not look as pretty or be as large as the commercially grown produce, but you won't get the added chemicals and you'll probably get more vitamins, minerals, and flavor.

Through the years, many clients have commented that they feel so much healthier following the Formula simply because they started eating fruits and vegetables again. Always check to see what's in season to add variety to your diet.

Try the delicious Summer Fresh Fruit Salad on the following page for a nutrient-packed Formula lunch.

Lunch	FORMULA 40-30-30 FAT FLUSH MEAL PLAN PERSONAL REQUIREMENTS*				
Summer Fresh Fruit Salad	A	B	C	D	E
Yogurt, fat-free, plain	4 oz.	5 oz.	5 oz.	8 oz.	10 oz.
Cottage cheese, 1% lowfat	½ cup	¾ cup	¾ cup	1 cup	1½ cups
Blueberries	¼ cup	½ cup	½ cup	½ cup	¾ cup
Peaches	¼ cup	½ cup	½ cup	½ cup	½ cup
Honeydew melon	½ cup	½ cup	½ cup	½ cup	½ cup
Macadamia nuts, chopped	1⅓ tbsp.	2 tbsp.	2 tbsp.	2½ tbsp.	3 tbsp.

DIRECTIONS: Blend yogurt and cottage cheese. Place in a bowl and top with fresh fruit and nuts.

For more than 200 personalized meals and recipes, including the Formula 40-30-30 Fat Flush Meals, refer to our book *The Formula*.

*To know your A, B, C, D, or E Meal Plan Personal Requirements, refer to Appendix A: The Formula Meal Plan Selection Chart.

73

MEASURE WHEN COOKING

◆

We like to encourage clients to measure their food when preparing a meal. An accurate kitchen scale is a good way to familiarize yourself with appropriate servings of protein. Four ounces of chicken will be a smaller portion than 4 ounces of fish, as chicken is more dense than most fish. If you require 35 grams of protein at dinner, a kitchen scale will prove valuable in helping you determine the correct amount required. After a few weeks of weighing, you will know amounts just by looking at them and you can put the scale away.

Have a complete set of measuring cups and spoons. If a meal calls for one cup of strawberries, measure the first few times so you know what a cup of strawberries looks like. After that, you will have a pretty good idea of the amount and no longer need to measure.

It is even more important to measure fat sources. One tablespoon of chopped macadamia nuts contains 6 grams of fat. One tablespoon of olive oil contains 14 grams of fat. Without actually measuring, you can dramatically affect the fat grams and calories of a meal if you guess wrong.

74

DON'T SHOP HUNGRY AND ALWAYS USE A SHOPPING LIST

Before heading off to the grocery store, be sure you have recently eaten one of your scheduled meals or snack. Studies have shown that hungry shoppers are more likely to purchase unnecessary and less nutritious foods. Eating a balanced meal every four to five hours helps to maintain stable blood sugar, eliminating hunger from meal to meal. If it's been a while since your last meal and it's time for your snack, have a 40-30-30 Nutrition Bar with a bottle of water while you are shopping.

Always prepare a shopping list. Research has shown that dieters who follow precise meal plans and use a shopping list lose 50% more weight than those who don't. Review the Formula meals and choose several favorites for the upcoming week. Look over the recipes and prepare your shopping list. Keep a running list that can be posted on the refrigerator and add items to it after the week's menus have been planned and whenever items are running low.

Shop primarily on the perimeter of the store, where you find produce, deli, dairy, fresh fish, and meats. It's best to completely avoid certain aisles. We seldom walk down the frozen foods aisle and don't even waste our time in the candy, cereal, cookie, cracker, and chip aisles.

We shop primarily at three stores: the closer chain grocery store, Costco for bulk foods, and the health food store. Because we don't go to Costco or the health food store as often, we keep a separate shopping list for bulk foods and specialty health food store items and vitamin supplements.

75

MAKE YOUR OWN DELICIOUS SALAD DRESSING

Many of the Formula dinner meals contain salads. Although lettuce is a minuscule part of the actual carbohydrates in the meal (2 cups of mixed salad greens contain 4 grams of carbohydrates), the salad becomes the vehicle for adding fat. Each Formula meal contains 30% of calories from fat. The fat slows the rate at which carbohydrates enter your bloodstream, cause the release of a hormone that signals your brain to stop eating, and provides the feeling of fullness while making food taste better.

Olive oil is the preferred source of oil when making salad dressings. It is a monounsaturated fat. Many of the recipes call for olive oil and vinegar salad dressing. Bottled olive oil and vinegar dressings typically provide about 4 grams of fat per tablespoon. It is important to measure the appropriate amount, rather than just pouring salad dressing on your salad. Our favorite bottled dressing is Newman's Own Balsamic Vinaigrette at 4.5 grams of fat per tablespoon. But Joyce's favorite homemade dressing is the one her mom always made when she was growing up. Her mom could make it perfectly just by pouring it directly on the salad greens and tossing. Joyce still measures.

Try these for a variety of delicious, heart-healthy dressings, each with only 4 grams of fat per tablespoon.

Mom's Olive Oil and Vinegar Salad Dressing

3 tablespoons olive oil

3 tablespoons red wine vinegar

3 tablespoons water

1 tablespoon fresh lemon juice

1½ teaspoons sugar or fructose

¼ teaspoon garlic salt

⅛ teaspoon salt

⅛ teaspoon ground black pepper

DIRECTIONS: Place all ingredients in a small glass jar or bottle and shake well. Variations include substituting 1 tablespoon red wine vinegar with balsamic vinegar and 1 clove fresh minced garlic for garlic salt and increase salt to ¼ teaspoon.

Honey Mustard Vinaigrette

3 tablespoons olive oil

3 tablespoons water

2 tablespoons fresh lemon juice

1 tablespoon red wine vinegar

1 teaspoon honey

2 teaspoons spicy brown mustard

½ teaspoon dried mustard powder

¼ teaspoon garlic

⅛ teaspoon salt

⅛ teaspoon pepper

DIRECTIONS: Place all ingredients in a small glass jar or bottle and shake well.

76

CONSIDER PEANUTS AND PEANUT BUTTER HIGH-FAT FOODS

Peanuts and peanut butter contain approximately 70% fat and should be considered high-fat foods, not high-protein. Peanuts aren't really even a nut; they are a legume, part of the bean family. Because they are a legume, many vegetarians think of peanuts and peanut butter as high-protein foods, but they are not. Two tablespoons of peanut butter or about 1 ounce of peanuts contain approximately 5 grams of carbohydrates (about 11% of the calories), 7 grams of low-quality protein (about 17% of the calories), and 14 grams of high-quality fat (about 73% of the calories). As you can see, even though peanuts and peanut butter contain a little protein, they contain more than 70% fat.

Also, the protein in peanuts and peanut butter is not a high-quality protein. It is very low in the essential amino acid methionine. In fact, peanuts and peanut butter have a usable protein score of only 41%. This means that for every 10 grams of protein you eat from peanuts and peanut butter, your body really uses only about 4 grams of it. So peanuts and peanut butter are not a great source of protein.

On the other hand, peanuts and peanut butter are a great source of "good fats." More than 50% of the fat from peanuts and peanut butter is from monounsaturated fat ("good fats").

We use peanuts and peanut butter in some of our Formula recipes as a source of good fat. When you are preparing your own favorite meals, consider peanuts and peanut butter as high-fat foods, not high-protein.

77

HAVE ONE-THIRD MORE CARBOHYDRATE THAN PROTEIN

The Formula is about balanced nutrition. A great way to help you always eat a balanced meal or snack is to simply remember to always eat one-third more carbohydrates than protein.

The Formula uses the revolutionary 40-30-30 balanced nutrition ratio. That means every meal should contain 40% of the total calories from carbohydrate, 30% from protein, and 30% from fat. Another way to think of it is to always have one-third more carbohydrates in a meal than protein. Since 1991, this simple but powerful 40-30-30 ratio has helped millions of people burn fat, lose weight, and feel and perform better.

Try using this method the next time you're in the grocery store in the yogurt section. A typical 6-ounce fruit yogurt has approximately 48 grams of carbohydrate, 10 grams of protein, and 2 grams of fat. That's almost five times more carbohydrate than protein. Most yogurts are high in carbohydrates because they are loaded with sugar to make them taste sweet. If a yogurt has 10 grams of protein, it should have only one-third more carbohydrates or 13 grams. Because carbohydrates and proteins each contain 4 calories per gram, the one-third more works for both the calories and the grams. So, when you are looking at any food to see if it is balanced, simply check out the protein first and the carbohydrates should be about one-third more.

This is a useful tip to help you understand balanced nutrition. We know that many people find it difficult to figure out how to do it on their own. Most people simply want to know what to eat. In *The Formula*, we show you exactly how to use yogurt as well as more than 200 meals and recipes designed for your personal requirements.

For a simple way to help keep your diet balanced and your body burning fat faster, always remember to have about one-third more carbohydrate than protein in a meal.

78

DON'T CARB-LOAD BEFORE YOU EXCERCISE

Exercise is a great way to burn calories and reduce body fat. But carbohydrate loading before you exercise may be decreasing your fat-burning potential. To maximize your body's natural ability to burn stored body fat and to get the most out of your workout, don't carbohydrate-load before you exercise.

One of the biggest fallacies in sports nutrition is that the body prefers to use carbohydrates for energy. This is simply not true. The body prefers to use fat for energy, stored body fat! But if you eat too many carbohydrates before you work out, you force your body to burn glucose for energy instead of stored body fat.

Carbohydrate loading before exercise makes absolutely no sense. Excess carbohydrates cause blood sugar to rise, stimulating the release of the hormone insulin. Insulin is your body's fat storage hormone. Excess insulin slows down your body's natural ability to access stored body fat for energy. Even worse, insulin converts the excess carbohydrates into fat.

Basically, by carbohydrate loading, you are minimizing your ability to burn fat during exercise. It's like taking two steps backwards even before you start exercising, simply because you carbohydrate-loaded. Years of hearing that carbohydrates give us energy had millions of people carbohydrate-loading before workouts. It's no wonder that many people were unhappy with their results. We have worked with thousands of people who were going to stop working out because they weren't seeing results. Many personal trainers were just as frustrated. But, once we explained that carbohydrate loading was the problem, they switched to the 40-30-30 nutrition solution and their workouts started to pay off.

To maximize the benefits of exercise, eat a balanced 40-30-30 snack before your workout instead of carbohydrate loading. Balanced nutrition will maintain stable blood sugar and insulin levels. Having a little protein in the snack will not only help your body build and repair muscle, which helps you burn fat faster, it will activate your fat-burning hormone glucagon, which helps your body burn fat even faster. Exercise works, but your diet controls how well it works.

79

DON'T SUFFER FROM LOW BLOOD SUGAR BLUES

◆

Many people suffer with symptoms of low blood sugar such as headaches, confusion and weakness, dizziness, tremors, irregular heartbeat, nervousness, and hunger. Normal blood sugar levels range between 70 and 120 milligrams per deciliter. Hypoglycemia is defined as abnormally low blood glucose concentration.

Hypoglycemia can occur when too many carbohydrates are eaten at a meal. Blood sugar levels surge, stimulating excess levels of insulin and increased production of adrenaline, causing nervousness followed by low blood sugar. For years, Joyce experienced hypoglycemic symptoms. Several hours after eating a high-carbohydrate breakfast, her blood sugar levels would drop, leaving her hungry, shaky, light-headed, and unable to concentrate. She relied on chocolate candy to raise blood sugar temporarily, relieving some of the symptoms. Her typical breakfast was a bowl of cereal with a small amount of milk and orange juice. When she ate donuts of any kind, her symptoms were intensified. But when she learned about the 40-30-30 Formula and the hormonal effects of a balanced meal, she ate breakfasts that stabilized blood sugar levels and her hypoglycemic symptoms disappeared. Her favorite breakfasts are either a 40-30-30 Balance

Bar with a small cup of decaffeinated coffee or the Oatmeal and Cottage Cheese Formula 40-30-30 Fat Flush breakfast.

For those with severe hypoglycemic symptoms, we recommend using the Formula 40-30-30 Fat Flush meals, those containing only low- to medium-glycemic carbohydrates. Eat your meal slowly, taking about 20 to 30 minutes if possible. Joyce cuts a 40-30-30 Balance Bar into small M&M-size pieces and nibbles on them. It just seems to work better eating it slowly.

80

INCLUDE OATMEAL
IN YOUR DIET

There's no better comfort food on a cold winter morning than a bowl of steaming hot oatmeal. But oatmeal with brown sugar, butter, and cream is not exactly a balanced meal. One cup of cooked oatmeal contains 25 grams of carbohydrates, but, with the addition of sugar, butter, and cream, you can make a heart-healthy breakfast not much better than two glazed donuts.

HIGH-FAT OATMEAL CEREAL

	Calories	Carbohydrates	Protein	Fat
1 cup cooked oatmeal	147	25.2 grams	6 grams	2.4 grams
1 tablespoon brown sugar	48	12	0	0
1 tablespoon butter	99	0	0	11
¼ cup half and half	70	2.6	2	6
Total grams		39.2	8	19.4
Calories per gram		×4	×4	×9
Total calories	364	157	32	175
Percentage of calories		43%	9%	48%

TWO GLAZED DONUTS

	Calories	Carbohydrates	Protein	Fat
Two Glazed Donuts	332	34 grams	4 grams	20 grams
Calories per gram		×4	×4	×9
Total calories	332	136	16	180
Percentage of calories		41%	5%	54%

Instant oatmeal sold in packets has been processed and is even worse. It will have a higher glycemic response than steel-cut, slow-cook oatmeal, and many have added sugar and flavors. A small, single-pack serving of instant, cinnamon-spice oatmeal breaks down this way:

INSTANT OATMEAL

	Calories	Carbohydrates	Protein	Fat
Instant Oatmeal	174	35 grams	4 grams	2 grams
Calories per gram		×4	×4	×9
Total calories	174	140	16	18
Percentage of calories		82%	9%	11%

Oatmeal can be a breakfast superfood when it's part of a balanced meal. This fiber-rich grain is a carbohydrate-dense food: ¼ cup dry, steel-cut oatmeal supplies 26 grams of carbohydrate, 4 grams of protein, and 2 grams of fat. By adding lowfat protein and quality fat, you can eat a heart-healthy balanced breakfast that can give you the comfort of knowing you are burning fat all morning.

Try warming yourself up in the morning with the following delicious oatmeal breakfast recipe. It is perfectly balanced with protein and fat. And it's not only good—it's good for you.

MEAL PLAN PERSONAL REQUIREMENTS*

Breakfast

Formula Oatmeal and Cream

	A	B	C	D	E
Oatmeal, cooked amount	½ cup	½ cup	¾ cup	1 cup	1 ⅓ cups
Cottage cheese, 2% lowfat	⅓ cup	⅓ cup	⅔ cup	¾ cup	1 cup
Brown sugar	1 tsp.	1 tsp.	1½ tsp.	2 tsp.	2 tsp.
Whipped butter	½ tsp.	½ tsp.	1 tsp.	1½ tsp.	1½ tsp.
Milk, 1% lowfat	3 tbsp.	3 tbsp.	3 tbsp.	¼ cup	¼ cup
Almonds, sliced	2 tsp.	2 tsp.	1 tbsp.	1⅓ tbsp.	1¾ tbsp.

DIRECTIONS: Cook oatmeal in water according to package directions. Blend in cottage cheese and top with brown sugar, butter, milk, and almonds. Cottage cheese melts and becomes very creamy. It can also be served on the side.

For more than 200 personalized meals and recipes, including the Formula 40-30-30 Fat Flush Meals, refer to our book *The Formula*.

*To know your A, B, C, D, or E Meal Plan Personal Requirements, refer to Appendix A: The Formula Meal Plan Selection Chart.

81

BOOST YOUR METABOLISM BY LIFTING WEIGHTS

Strength training with the Formula will boost your metabolism by providing the carbohydrates, protein, and fat necessary to build lean muscle mass. Exercise is a critical part of any weight-loss program. It improves insulin metabolism, burns more calories, reduces abdominal fat, and increases the fitness of your heart, lungs, circulation, and metabolism. Exercise increases energy levels and lowers blood sugar and insulin levels, thus reducing your risk for diabetes.

Strength training is now being thought of as potentially more beneficial than aerobic exercise for improving bone density, strengthening the heart, and reducing such risk factors for heart disease as insulin resistance, high blood pressure, and obesity. Weight training prevents muscle loss due to aging, increases muscle protein synthesis, builds strength, and improves cells' metabolism. Scientists have learned that increasing strength can dramatically improve your quality of life. A strong body will give you the muscle power to help you stay active and physical with less effort.

But the best benefit of strength training is that it helps to greatly increase your metabolism so that your body will burn more stored fat and calories, even while resting. Bodybuilders have known for more than 50 years now that building muscle through weight training (or other strength exercise) is the fastest way to boost your metabolism and help your body burn fat faster, even while you sleep.

Try lifting some weights or incorporating some other type of strength exercises into your exercise program. It will do your body good.

82

TEACH YOUR FAVORITE RESTAURANT HOW TO MAKE 40-30-30 FORMULA MEALS

If you have a favorite bagel shop, sandwich shop, or restaurant that you stop in often, you can teach them how to make 40-30-30 Formula meals. Sandwich shops and local restaurants love their regular customers. In fact, it's their regular customers who keep them in business. Many of our clients have told us how they learned to order 40-30-30 meals from their favorite restaurants.

A good friend of ours used to buy a bagel with cream cheese and coffee every morning from the neighborhood bagel shop. After learning about the Formula, he continues to order the bagel, but has them add sliced turkey and lowfat cream cheese. He says they have it waiting for him Monday through Friday, 8:00 A.M., like clockwork.

We have a favorite Mexican restaurant we enjoy. Whenever they see Joyce, they comment "No beans, no rice." They make her a perfect 40-30-30 Chicken Burrito with a flour tortilla, shredded chicken, salsa, cilantro, hot peppers, and a side order of sour cream or guacamole.

We've heard from clients around the country who had their favorite Formula Smoothie added to the menu at the local juice bar. In fact, many gyms and health food stores with juice bars offer 40-30-30 Formula Shakes. One woman had the cottage cheese, fruit, and nuts Formula 40-30-30 Fat Flush breakfast added to the menu at her local small-town restaurant.

Talk to the owner of your favorite restaurants and you may be pleasantly surprised to find your 40-30-30 Formula meal show up on the menu.

83

MAKE E-SIZE SHAKES FOR AFTER-SCHOOL SNACKS

When your kids come home from school and they are starving for a snack, make sure that it's balanced. It's easy to see why childhood obesity and diabetes are on the rise. Children are eating and drinking more carbohydrates than ever, afterschool snacks are notoriously unsupervised, and many children participate in little or no exercise. But you can begin to take control of your children's eating habits by removing the junk food from your house. Don't buy cookies, soda, chips, and other foods you know are unhealthy. Instead, keep low-glycemic fruits and protein on hand or make the 40-30-30 Smoothies.

One of our clients makes a blenderful of her son's favorite Formula Smoothie, the Banana Peanut Butter Smoothie. She told us she has the reputation of making the best afterschool milk shakes. Her son and his two best friends split a blenderful of Formula Smoothies before hopping on their bikes or playing sports. Her son used to suffer from energy slumps after school. The high-carbohydrate cookies and milk snack only made matters worse and he was gaining weight.

When she switched to the Formula Shake, his energy improved and he leaned up.

Try making the E size shake for your kids and their friends. The extra large E size shake can be split into three snack-size servings. You might just become the coolest mom in the neighborhood.

Snack

KIDS' FAVORITE

Banana Peanut Butter Smoothie

	MEAL PLAN PERSONAL REQUIREMENTS*				
	A	B	C	D	E
Banana, medium	⅔	1	1	1⅓	1¾
Milk, 1% lowfat	⅔ cup	¾ cup	¾ cup	1 cup	1 cup
Peanut butter, natural	2½ tsp.	1⅓ tbsp.	1⅓ tbsp.	1¾ tbsp.	2⅓ tbsp.
Pure whey protein powder	10 grams	20 grams	20 grams	25 grams	33 grams

DIRECTIONS: Combine all ingredients in a blender and process until smooth. Use frozen bananas for a thicker smoothie. *Note*: For more information on pure whey protein, please refer to Appendix C: Special Ingredients.

For more than 200 personalized meals and recipes, including the Formula 40-30-30 Fat Flush Meals, refer to our book *The Formula*.

*To know your A, B, C, D, or E Meal Plan Personal Requirements, refer to Appendix A: The Formula Meal Plan Selection Chart.

84

UNDERSTAND THAT NOT ALL PROTEINS ARE CREATED EQUAL

Throughout this book and in *The Formula*, we emphasize the importance of eating quality protein every time you eat. Quality protein in a meal stimulates the release of the hormone glucagon, one of the body's most powerful fat-burning hormones. Glucagon mobilizes the release of stored body fat to be used for energy. The protein and fat in a meal help regulate the hormones that can help you burn fat faster.

The quality of protein is determined by two factors: its digestibility and its amino acid profile. Beans, for example, contain protein and carbohydrates. They are also high in fiber. The fiber wraps around the protein chains, making it difficult to use the amino acids and, therefore, difficult to digest. Beans are also an incomplete source of protein, lacking in some of the essential amino acids. Protein nutrition is all about balance. All of the amino acids must be present in the right balance for the body to use the protein fully. It doesn't matter how much protein a food contains; if that food is low in just one amino acid, your body can use only the amount of the lowest amino acid found in that food. This is known as the rate-limiting amino acid. The quality of protein food is limited to the lowest amount of essential amino acid that is in that food. Three ounces of black beans contain about 6 grams of protein, but they are very low in the essential amino acid methionine. They have a usable protein score of only 50%. That means that for every 10 grams of black bean protein that you eat, you can use only about 5 grams of protein. Black beans are a nutritious food, but use them as a carbohydrate source, not a protein.

In general, most plant proteins are more difficult to digest and have poor amino acid profiles compared to animal proteins. This is not to say that you should eat only animal proteins or that you should avoid plant proteins. Good nutrition is a balance. We always consider both factors when designing Formula meals.

Here is a list of some common protein foods and their Usable Protein Score. Use this as a guide to help you prepare high-quality protein meals. The egg is considered one of nature's most perfect protein foods because of its ease of digestion and protein usability.

COMMON PROTEIN FOODS

Food	Amount	Protein Grams	Usable Protein Score	Limiting Amino Acid
Eggs	1 whole	6	101%	None
Cottage cheese, lowfat	½ cup	14	93%	Trytophan @ 93%
Chicken breast, skinless	3 ounces	26	83%	Phenylalanine @ 83%
Turkey, skinless	3 ounces	25	83%	Phenylalanine @ 83%
Salmon	3 ounces	23	81%	Phenylalanine @ 81%
Beef tenderloin	3 ounces	21	81%	Phenylalanine @ 83%
White rice	3 ounces	1.5	77%	Lysine @ 77%

Black beans	3 ounces	6	50%	Methionine @ 50%
Tofu, firm	3 ounces	13	43%	Methionine @ 43%
Almonds	3 ounces	17	38%	Methionine @ 38%

Make sure your meals contain adequate amounts of high-quality, easy-to-digest protein.

85

TAKE A 40-30-30 NUTRITION BAR THE NEXT TIME YOU SKI

You can improve your performance in any sport with balanced nutrition. If you want to keep your energy levels up and improve endurance, take along a 40-30-30 Nutrition Bar the next time you go skiing. Forget those high-carbohydrate bars and the bonk that can come from them, and start using a more balanced approach.

When we were first introduced to the 40-30-30 zone diet in 1991, we thought we knew it all. Like most athletes, we were following a high-carbohydrate, lowfat diet. After reviewing the research on the importance of balanced nutrition, we were convinced that 40-30-30 could be one of the greatest breakthroughs in sports nutrition. From a performance standpoint, the research was very clear. Either eat lots of carbohydrates and burn only glucose for energy, or eat a balance of carbohydrates, protein, and fat to stabilize blood sugar and tap into stored fat for energy, while sparing glucose for your brain and muscles.

We are both hard-training athletes as well as avid skiers. After changing our diet to the 40-30-30 ratio and seeing great results, we started using the world's first 40-30-30 Nutrition Bars. We will never forget how much better we skied the first time we tried one of the 40-30-30 Nutrition Bars.

We had lots of energy, better oxygen uptake, less lactic acid buildup in our legs, and were able to ski all-out from 9:00 A.M. to 1:00 P.M.

We have been skiing many times since those original days. We always take a 40-30-30 Nutrition Bar and are amazed at how good we feel and ski. After helping more than 500,000 people use this technology, we are convinced now more than ever that 40-30-30 is one of the greatest breakthroughs ever in nutrition. Athletes in every sport used to rely on carbohydrates for energy, but new research in sports nutrition and fat utilization has changed all that.

There are many companies making 40-30-30 nutrition bars. Listed below are a few of the bars that we use and recommend:

- Balance Bar by the Balance Bar Company
- Ironman Triathlon Bar by Twin Laboratories, Inc.
- PR Bar by PR Nutrition Inc.
- 40-30-30 Bar by Trader Joe's

40-30-30 Nutrition Bars now come in many flavors and taste great. Try one the next time you go skiing or participate in any sport.

86

LOWERING CALORIES
ISN'T THE ANSWER

The amount of calories and the balance of carbohydrate, protein, and fat they contain will ultimately determine how successful you are with any weight-loss or nutrition program. It is important that you understand that simply lowering calories isn't the answer to reducing body fat.

Throughout this book and *The Formula* we have explained the importance of balanced nutrition. The balance of calories is as important as the amount of calories when it comes to burning fat, losing weight, and performing better.

Many experts believe that a calorie is a calorie, and to lose weight, you must simply eat fewer calories. They obviously can't see the forest for the trees. Although they may be somewhat correct in saying that when you lower calories you can lose weight, it usually is muscle weight. But, if your goal is to lose *fat weight* while maintaining muscle, then the balance of carbohydrate, protein, and fat and adequate calorie consumption become critical and far more important than simply lowering calories.

Low-calorie diets that are high in carbohydrates and low in fat have been proven to fail. They fail because they do not contain adequate protein to maintain and build muscle (remember, the more muscle you have, the more fat and calories you can burn). Low-calorie diets also do not contain enough "good fat" to help keep blood sugar stable and control insulin.

A 1,500-calorie diet that is high in carbohydrates and low in fat will generate a completely different hormonal response from a 1,500-calorie balanced diet of carbohydrate, protein, and fat. Your hormonal response to your meals will determine how efficiently your body burns or stores fat.

So remember: The balance of the calories you eat is far more important than simply lowering calories. To maximize fat loss, maintain lean muscle mass, and perform better, eat an adequate amount of calories in the ratio of 40% carbohydrates, 30% protein, and 30% fat at every meal. It's what we call "the Formula."

87

BE
PREPARED

◆

Just like a good Boy Scout, if you want to get the best results when following the Formula, you must be prepared. So plan ahead, and when you do your grocery shopping, shop for at least one week's worth of groceries.

By planning ahead and shopping for all of your favorite foods, you will be well prepared to successfully follow the Formula for a lifetime. Here are additional ideas to help you be better prepared:

- Stock up on frozen bags of skinless, boneless chicken breast. Most of the warehouse-type stores sell large bags of frozen, skinless chicken breast. Some even have precooked chicken strips.

- Buy the large-size bag of gourmet salad greens or romaine lettuce. This is one our favorite convenience foods because we eat salads so often. You can also buy these at many of the warehouse stores.

- Stock up on your favorite packaged or canned goods. We always keep plenty of our favorite foods around, like macadamia nuts, fructose, and canned tuna, peaches, pears, tomatoes, and black beans.

- Brew a pot of decaffeinated tea and keep a pitcher of cold iced tea in the refrigerator ready for lunch or dinner.

- Buy eggs in cartons of 18 so you always have plenty on hand.

- Keep a large bowl of 40-30-30 Nutrition Bars on your kitchen counter. Your family can easily grab a bar for snacks. Buy the bars by the box and save money.

- Keep this book and *The Formula* out on your kitchen counter. Of course, this is our favorite recommendation. Hundreds of our clients have told us they keep our books displayed in their kitchens. They place it on a book stand for easy access to personalized meals and recipes. When your nutrition coaches are right there in your kitchen watching you, you always have a reminder to keep your meals balanced.

Follow this advice to help you be more prepared in your kitchen.

88

TRY GENE'S POWER PACK FOR THE ULTIMATE POWER LUNCH

I f you want to experience the ultimate edge at work or anytime, blend up Gene's Power Pack Smoothie.

Gene has been involved in sports nutrition, weight training, and bodybuilding since the early 1970s. He has always been a fan of protein shakes to help boost overall performance. For years, he drank the original Power Pack shake from one of the first juice bars in Ocean Beach, California. The "original" was loaded with bananas, juice, protein powder, and bee pollen. It was also very high in carbohydrates and contained very little fat. We modified and improved that shake into what it is today: Gene's Power Pack. It is 40-30-30 and still fortified with bee pollen. It contains both high- and low-glycemic carbohydrates from bananas and strawberries, whey protein, Vitamin C, B Vitamins, minerals, and flax oil. Gene swears that it makes his cells come alive. Try it sometime for lunch and feel the power.

Lunch

Gene's Power Pack

	MEAL PLAN PERSONAL REQUIREMENTS*				
	A	B	C	D	E
Banana, medium	⅓ cup	½ cup	½ cup	¾ cup	1 cup
Strawberries, frozen	1 cup	1 cup	1 cup	1½ cups	1⅔ cups
Milk, 1% lowfat	½ cup	1 cup	1 cup	1 cup	1½ cups
Pure whey protein powder	15 grams	20 grams	20 grams	30 grams	35 grams
Bee pollen	1 tsp.	1 tsp.	1 tsp.	1½ tsp.	1½ tsp.
Emer`gen-C packet	1	1	1	1	1
Flax oil	½ tbsp.	¾ tbsp.	¾ tbsp.	1¼ tbsp.	1⅓ tbsp.

DIRECTIONS: Combine all ingredients in a blender and process until smooth. Use frozen bananas for a thicker shake. Bee pollen, Emer`gen-C, and flax oil can be found in health food stores. *Note:* For more information on pure whey protein, please refer to Appendix C: Special Ingredients.

For more than 200 personalized meals and recipes, including the Formula 40-30-30 Fat Flush Meals, refer to our book *The Formula*.

*To know your A, B, C, D, or E Meal Plan Personal Requirements, refer to Appendix A: The Formula Meal Plan Selection Chart.

89

DRINK YOUR VEGGIES

t can sometimes be hard to include vegetables in your diet. One way to make sure you are getting enough vegetables is to drink a veggie smoothie.

Now, we know what you're thinking: How can a vegetable smoothie taste good enough to drink? Well, through trial and error we have designed a veggie smoothie tasty enough to get our seal of approval. We call it the Salad Smoothie. It is one of Gene's favorites and one he often drinks after a hard workout.

Try the Salad Smoothie snack recipe on the following page for a delicious way to include more vegetables in your diet.

Snack

Salad Smoothie

FORMULA 40-30-30 FAT FLUSH
MEAL PLAN PERSONAL REQUIREMENTS*

	A	B	C	D	E
Fresh green juice (celery, spinach, cucumbers, lettuce, parsley, kale, wheat grass, greens)	8 ounces	8 ounces	8 ounces	8 ounces	16 ounces
Emer`gen-C packet	1	1	1	1	1
Peaches, frozen	½ cup	½ cup	½ cup	½ cup	1 cup
Pure whey protein powder	15 grams	15 grams	15 grams	15 grams	30 grams
Bee pollen	1 tsp.	1 tsp.	1 tsp.	1 tsp.	1½ tsp.
Flax oil	½ tbsp.	½ tbsp.	½ tbsp.	½ tbsp.	1 tbsp.

DIRECTIONS: Combine all ingredients in a blender and process until smooth. Juice your own greens or buy fresh bottled green juice at the health food store. Look for bottled juice without any fruit juices added. Emer`gen-C can be found in health food stores and is a powdered packet of Vitamin C with minerals and B Vitamins. Bee pollen and flax oil can be found in health food stores. *Note:* For more information on pure whey protein, please refer to Appendix C: Special Ingredients.

For more than 200 personalized meals and recipes, including the Formula 40-30-30 Fat Flush Meals, refer to our book *The Formula.*

*To know your A, B, C, D, or E Meal Plan Personal Requirements, refer to Appendix A: The Formula Meal Plan Selection Chart.

90

TRY PITA POCKET BREAD

When preparing sandwiches, use whole-grain pita pocket bread as an alternative to regular breads. Whole-grain pita pockets are a good source of fiber, are lower glycemic, and contain more protein than regular bread. In fact, one whole-grain pita pocket contains about 6 grams of protein. You can stuff them full of sliced deli meats, chicken, or tuna salad, add sprouts, tomato, cucumber slices, and some mayonnaise or avocado. Eat it with fresh fruit and you have a great-tasting, balanced 40-30-30 Formula meal.

Try the lunch recipe on the following page and you'll see that whole wheat pita pockets are a great bread alternative.

MEAL PLAN PERSONAL REQUIREMENTS*

Lunch

Deli Salad Pita Pocket

	A	B	C	D	E
Deli-style tuna or chicken salad with full-fat mayonnaise	4 oz.	5 oz.	5 oz.	7 oz.	9 oz.
Pita bread, whole wheat	½	¾	¾	1	1
Apple	½ medium	½ medium	½ medium	1 medium	1 large

DIRECTIONS: Purchase tuna or chicken salad made with full-fat mayonnaise from a deli. Place in pita pocket and serve with fruit.

For more than 200 personalized meals and recipes, including the Formula 40-30-30 Fat Flush Meals, refer to our book *The Formula*.

*To know your A, B, C, D, or E Meal Plan Personal Requirements, refer to Appendix A: The Formula Meal Plan Selection Chart.

91

COOK A
WHOLE TURKEY

One of our favorite recommendations is to cook a whole turkey. It's a great way to always have ready-to-eat, high-quality protein around that you can use for many types of meals and recipes. After cooking the turkey, let it cool. Slice the meat and package it in 4- to 6-ounce packages. Keep a few packages in the refrigerator and freeze the rest. Now you have precooked protein whenever you need it. Also, freeze the turkey carcass and use it for delicious homemade turkey soup.

Turkey is one the best proteins you can eat. It is high-quality protein and very easy to digest. Four ounces of roasted, skinless, white turkey meat has approximately 0 grams of carbohydrate, 25 grams of protein, and only about 2 grams of fat. Turkey is also a great source of Vitamins B-12, niacin, and B-6. Cooking a whole turkey is very economical, especially when you buy it during the holidays. Compared to other proteins, turkey is quite a bargain.

We began cooking whole turkeys in 1985 when we were training for mixed-pairs bodybuilding competitions. We would cook a whole turkey about every two to three weeks and loved having this convenient protein source available for making quick and easy meals. When we traveled, we would take along a couple of bags of frozen turkey with some apples or oranges and almonds. It was great to always have a Formula 40-30-30 Fat Flush meal available.

One of our favorite ways to cook a turkey is to use a cooking bag. You can find cooking bags in your local grocery store. You will love having this economical, convenient, and delicious protein food available to help you make quick and easy 40-30-30 Formula meals.

Oven-Bag Roasted Turkey

Purchase a whole turkey and turkey-size oven bags. Preheat oven to 350°F. Remove the skin and cut off any visible fat from the turkey. For added flavor, empty cavity and fill with one chopped onion, a celery stalk, parsley, and a few cloves of garlic. Add 1 tablespoon flour to oven bag and shake to coat.

Place the turkey inside the bag and place in a large roasting pan. Close bag with nylon tie and cut slits in the top of the bag as directed on the box. Cook according to chart for correct size and time. Remove from oven when done and let stand for at least 20 minutes before carving.

Note: You can also substitute a whole chicken for the turkey if you prefer.

92

LEARN HOW TO
EAT FAST FOOD

As nutrition coaches, one of the most common questions we get is: "Can I eat fast food and still follow the 40-30-30 Formula?" The short answer is yes. But, because typical fast food is so high in fat as well as high in high-glycemic carbohydrates, your choices at most fast-food restaurants are somewhat limited.

Here are several ideas to help you follow the 40-30-30 Formula when eating at fast-food restaurants:

- *Grilled chicken breast sandwich:* Almost all fast-food restaurants offer a grilled chicken breast sandwich. Order it without the cheese or mayonnaise or it will be too high in fat. Have it with a side green salad with 1 tablespoon of salad dressing and an iced tea.

- *Extra meat sandwiches:* Because meat is more expensive than all of the other ingredients on a sandwich, most sandwich restaurants put very little meat in their sandwiches. Order a turkey or chicken sandwich with extra meat on sourdough bread. Add sliced avocado, mustard, and extra vegetable fixings. Have it with mineral water or iced tea. If a thick roll or bun is used, ask that they pull out some of the middle of the roll to reduce some of the high-glycemic carbo-hydrates that are in the roll.

- *Chicken Caesar salads:* Many fast-food restaurants offer premade chicken Caesar salads. You can also find them at grocery stores. Have the salad with croutons or a small roll with bottled water or an iced tea. To convert it into a Formula 40-30-30 Fat Flush meal, avoid the croutons or roll and have the salad with an apple.

- *Wendy's chili:* This is one of Joyce's favorite fast-food meals, especially in the colder months. Wendy's chili is almost a perfect 40-30-30, so have it with an iced tea, mineral water, or a diet soda. *Note:* Avoid adding crackers or the Frostie.

Throughout this book and *The Formula* we have tried to be your nutrition coaches and teach you the importance of following a balanced diet. We always encourage our clients to eat healthy, fresh, balanced meals. We have provided you with hundreds of meals and recipes to easily prepare your own balanced 40-30-30 Formula meals. But sometimes, because of hectic schedules, it can be hard to find the time to make your own meals and you are forced to eat out. When you don't have the time to make your own meals, knowing how to choose balanced fast food can make it a good choice.

93

USE AVOCADO IN YOUR MEALS

Avocados are one of the most misunderstood of all foods. Most people think of avocados as "bad" because they are so high in fat. But a little avocado can and should be part of everyone's diet.

One-fourth of an avocado has approximately 4 grams of carbohydrate, 1 gram of protein, and 8 grams of fat. About 80% of the calories in an avocado come from fat, so yes, they are, in fact, very high in fat. But the fat in avocados is primarily monounsaturated, the good type of fat. In fact, along with macadamia nuts, olives, and olive oil, avocados are one of the best sources for monounsaturated fats.

Like everything in nutrition, it's all about moderation and balance. There really is no food that is off limits, as long as it is used in moderation and balance, and that includes the use of high-fat foods like avocados. Because they are so high in fat, you will always want to use a small amount of avocado in your meals and recipes. Just remember to use avocados as a good source of fat and use small amounts.

Here a a few ways you can include avocado in your diet:

- *Sandwiches:* Add a couple of slices of avocado on your sandwich instead of mayonnaise or cheese. One of Gene's favorite ways to use avocado is on a roast reef sandwich on rye bread with mustard and sliced avocado.

- *Burritos and fajitas:* Instead of sour cream or excess cheese, use sliced avocado in burritos and fajitas.

- *Salads:* Go easy on some of the dressing that you would normally use and instead, add a few slices of avocado to your favorite salads.

- *On the side:* Whenever you might be a little low in fat in a meal or recipe, add a slice of avocado on the side to help balance.

Remember: Even though avocados are high in fat, it is classified as good fat and can and should be used as part of your balanced Formula diet.

94

DISCARD SOME OF THE MIDDLE OF THE BREAD

Here is a great tip, especially for bread lovers: Pull out some of the middle of the bread and discard it before eating buns, rolls, bagels, or French bread.

This is one of our favorite tips and one that Joyce has been using for years. Most rolls contain very high amounts of very-high-glycemic carbohydrates. Most breads are also made from very-high-glycemic white flour. White flour is rated at close to 100 on the glycemic scale, almost the same as pure sugar. This means that bread can increase your blood sugar just as fast as pure sugar. To help lower the carbohydrate content, simply pull out some of the middle of the roll and discard it.

This method works great for bagels. One of Gene's favorite lunches when we are traveling is a whole wheat turkey bagel sandwich. He asks to have the soft middle of the bagel removed and orders it with extra meat (at least 4 ounces) and extra tomatoes, cucumber, sprouts, and avocado. A small frozen bagel, 3½ -inch diameter, contains about 30 grams of carbohydrate, and larger bagels found in your local deli or bagel shop can contain as many as 50 to 60 carbohydrates. If you are using large bagels, 4½- to 5-inch diameter, you can also carefully slice the bagel horizontally in thirds or even fourths and use only 2 slices to reduce the calories before making a sandwich.

When eating French bread, slice horizontally and remove as much of the soft middle as possible, leaving the crusty top and bottom. We actually like it better without the middle and we always feel better for not eating it.

If you are going to eat bread, it's better to remove the soft middle rather than have it end up storing as fat on your soft middle.

95

OVO-LACTO VEGETARIAN DIETS WORK BEST

We have worked with thousands of individuals who considered themselves vegetarians. But many of them were not really vegetarians. Most simply did not eat beef, but would eat other animal proteins. For the few who did follow vegetarian diets, we saw the best results when they followed an ovo-lacto vegetarian diet.

There are several types of vegetarian diets. The three most popular are vegan, lacto vegetarian, and ovo-lacto vegetarian. A vegan, or strict vegetarian diet, eliminates all animal products. The problem is that it is very hard to balance vegan meals with high-quality, easy-to-digest protein. Unless a vegan eats a lot of tofu or tempeh at every meal, the diet will always be too high in carbohydrates and too low in protein.

Lacto vegetarian diets eliminate any type of meat and fish but allow dairy foods like cottage cheese. Lacto vegetarian diets are easier to balance than vegan diets. With the addition of dairy foods like lowfat cheeses and lowfat cottage cheese in meals along with tofu and tempeh, it is easier to supply adequate amounts of high-quality, easy-to-digest protein.

Ovo-lacto vegetarian diets eliminate any type of animal meats, including fish, but allow dairy products and eggs. In our opinion, this is the best of the three types of vegetarian diets to follow, because it is easy to balance with carbohydrates, proteins, and fat. Dairy and eggs are not only an excellent source of high-quality, easy-to-digest protein, they are delicious foods to include in your diet. Ovo-lacto vegetarian diets are less restrictive and it's easy to get adequate amounts of protein.

The Formula can work with any type of specialty diet, including vegetarian diets. Some types are just a little harder to keep balanced than others. If you want to follow a vegetarian diet, we recommend following an ovo-lacto vegetarian diet.

96

CONTROL THE CALORIES
IN A MEAL

◆

New research has confirmed what bodybuilders have known for years: that eating small calorie-controlled meals several times per day will help boost your metabolism and burn fat faster than eating large, infrequent meals. We have seen our clients get better results when they eat three meals a day plus one or two snacks, and when they keep their largest meals around 500 calories or fewer.

By eating smaller, more frequent meals you can help stabilize blood sugar. Stable blood sugar controls the release of the hormone insulin and allows you to burn stored body fat for energy. There are two ways to stimulate insulin with food: by eating too many carbohydrates in a meal, and by eating too many calories at one time. By following the balanced 40-30-30 Formula ratio and eating adequate calories for your specific requirements, you can help keep blood sugar and insulin levels balanced and burn fat faster.

Eating small, frequent meals also helps keep hunger in check. Small frequent meals keep your appetite controlled so you are less likely to overeat or binge on sweets. Eating balanced, small, frequent meals every four to five hours can help you maintain and build lean muscle mass. The more muscle you have, the faster your metabolism will be and the more fat and calories you will burn, 24 hours per day, 7 days per week.

For most people, 500 to 550 calories should be the maximum number of calories eaten at any meal. Breakfast and snacks should contain fewer. Very hard-training athletes can eat slightly more than 500 calories per meal. Because hard-training athletes' nutrient requirements can be much greater than the average person's, several meals on The Formula E plan are slightly larger than 600 calories.

For the best results, eat smaller meals several times a day and keep meals around 500 calories or fewer.

MEAL PLANNER MACRONUTRIENT CHART

Listed below are the total grams of carbohydrate, protein, fat, and calories for each meal plan. The meal plans have been tailored for individual requirements based on sex, weight, and activity level. To determine which meal plan is right for you, refer to the *The Formula Meal Plan Selection Chart* in the Appendix. Each meal and snack contains the 40-30-30 ratio, which provides 40% of its total calories from carbohydrate, 30% from protein, and 30% from fat.

PERSONAL MEAL PLANNER

Breakfast	A	B	C	D	E
Carbohydrate grams	20	20	33	47	53
Protein grams	15	15	25	35	40
Fat grams	6	6	11	13	18
Calories	194	194	331	445	534

Lunch					
Carbohydrate grams	27	40	40	53	66
Protein grams	20	30	30	40	50
Fat grams	9	14	14	18	22
Calories	269	406	406	534	662

Snacks					
Carbohydrate grams	20	20	20	20	40
Protein grams	15	15	15	15	30
Fat grams	6	6	6	6	12
Calories	194	194	194	194	388

Dinner					
Carbohydrate grams	40	47	53	53	66
Protein grams	30	35	40	40	50
Fat grams	14	15	18	18	22
Calories	406	463	534	534	662

Daily Totals					
Carbohydrate grams	106	126	146	173	226
Protein grams	80	95	110	130	170
Fat grams	35	42	48	57	75
Calories	1,063	1,257	1,465	1,707	2,246

97

SPLURGE ON VACATION

◇

An amazing thing happens when you get your diet balanced and improve your health: Your body becomes much more efficient at burning fat and calories for energy. When you have been following a balanced diet and have all of your muscles working efficiently, you have turned your body into an efficient fat-burning machine. The Formula and exercise can help you build and maintain lean muscle mass. The more muscle you have, the more fat and calories you can burn for energy.

After you have been following the Formula for a few months and you are in your fat-burning zone, try splurging on anything you like when you go on vacation. You will see that it helps keep you motivated by not depriving you of something special when you go to exciting new places. Many of our clients found that after a couple of high-carbohydrate treats, they actually preferred to follow a healthy balanced 40-30-30 diet for most of their trip because it made them feel better. But the most amazing thing is that once you have been following the Formula for a while and you have become more fit, your metabolism works more efficiently. We have seen that you can continue to burn fat and lose weight even while you are eating anything you want.

Two of our clients had been following the Formula program for about two months. They both wanted to lose fat and to get into shape for an upcoming vacation. Using body fat testing at our clinic, we saw that the man lost about 15 pounds of pure fat and gained 5 pounds of muscle. The women lost about 10 pounds of pure fat and gained 3 pounds of muscle. They were both completely happy with their results and were looking forward to a great vacation. When they returned, they were shocked to find that they had both actually lost a few more pounds of fat, even though they did absolutely no formal exercise and ate anything they wanted. We explained to them that their bodies were simply more fit and healthier and they were able to continue burning fat even though they were splurging on drinks and desserts.

So go ahead and splurge. It can help keep you motivated and can rev up your metabolism to help you burn fat faster.

98

LEARN HOW
TO JUICE

I f you are going to juice and follow the 40-30-30 Formula nutrition program successfully, you need to learn how to juice correctly. Most juice drinks are loaded with high amounts of carbohydrates. Basically, they contain just as much as or even more sugar than many soft drinks. A 12-ounce serving of carrot juice contains about 32 grams of carbohydrates. The carbohydrates from carrots are also very high-glycemic, which means they will elevate blood sugar.

Many of the popular juice bars also add frozen yogurt to their juice drinks. We have seen drinks containing more than 100 grams of carbohydrate in a single serving! If you want to stop burning fat and gain weight, a high-carbohydrate juice drink is just the ticket.

But if you want to juice and maximize your body's natural ability to burn stored body fat, try these simple recommendations the next time you order a juice drink:

- Choose a low-glycemic juice like peach, blueberry, or strawberry.
- Don't add frozen yogurt.

- Have 1 to 2 scoops of protein powder added to the shake (equal to 15 to 30 grams of protein).
- Include some fat from nuts or flaxseed oil.

These simple recommendations can help make juicing much more balanced and keep you on the path to fat-burning success.

99

ALWAYS HAVE SOME COOKED LOW-FAT PROTEIN IN YOUR REFRIGERATOR

Make following the Formula easier by always having some ready-to-eat, low-fat protein in your refrigerator or pantry.

Many protein foods need to be cooked before you can eat them. This makes protein the least convenient macronutrient to keep on hand. But by planning ahead, you can stock your kitchen and always be able to make a balanced 40-30-30 Formula meal.

Remember these ideas when planning your shopping list:

- Buy frozen or precooked chicken breast. Keep it on hand for chicken salads and many other Formula recipes.

- Hard-boil a dozen eggs. Peel them as needed and discard the appropriate number of yolks to reduce the fat.

- Have sliced deli-style turkey, chicken, lean beef, or lean ham around for sandwiches and salads.

- Keep lowfat cottage cheese on hand. Look at the date on the bottom of the container for the freshest you can find.

- Make extra grilled or smoked salmon. When salmon goes on sale at your local grocery store, fire up the grill and make extra for salads, sandwiches, and other recipes.

- Keep several cans or bags of tuna in your pantry. They are great for a quick tuna salad.

These are just a few ideas to help you get stocked up on protein. When you're out of protein, you're out of balance.

Here is a Hoagie Sandwich dinner recipe that incorporates this tip. Try it some evening for dinner.

Dinner

Hoagie Sandwich

	MEAL PLAN PERSONAL REQUIREMENTS*				
	A	B	C	D	E
Hoagie Sandwich (recipe below)	1½ slices	1¾ slices	2 slices	2 slices	2⅓ slices
Dill pickle	½	¾	1	1	1¾

HOAGIE SANDWICH RECIPE:

1 whole French bread loaf, 14–15 inches long, white or whole wheat

1 pound deli-style turkey breast

¼ pound deli-style, lowfat Swiss cheese

2 cups shredded lettuce

2 whole tomatoes, thinly sliced

½ sweet onion, thinly sliced

½ green bell pepper, thinly sliced

¾ avocado, sliced

2 tablespoons mustard

2 tablespoons Italian salad dressing, full-fat

RECIPE DIRECTIONS: Slice French bread in half horizontally and hollow out both halves by discarding the soft inside bread. Fill one half with turkey and cheese slices. Top with shredded lettuce and thinly sliced tomato, onion, and green pepper. Spread the avocado evenly in other half. Spread with mustard and drizzle with Italian dressing. Place both halves together and slice into 8 even portions to serve.

DIRECTIONS: Serve Hoagie Sandwich with dill pickle.

For more than 200 personalized meals and recipes, including the Formula 40-30-30 Fat Flush Meals, refer to our book *The Formula*.

*To know your A, B, C, D, or E Meal Plan Personal Requirements, refer to Appendix A: The Formula Meal Plan Selection Chart.

100

CLOSE IS
GOOD ENOUGH

When following the Formula, your meals don't have to contain a perfect 40-30-30 ratio to work. Close is good enough. Throughout this book and *The Formula*, we have explained the importance of balanced nutrition and using the 40-30-30 ratio as a guide when designing meals. Our books provide more than 200 meals and recipes that are delicious and easy for you to prepare. We did all the math for you.

When you begin to design your own meals, if they aren't exactly perfect, don't worry. You don't even have to count grams, calories, or food blocks. If you have been following the meals in our books, you will have learned by example. If you are served a meal with very little protein, don't eat many carbohydrates. If you are eating dinner at a friend's house and everything is swimming in butter and oil, eat around it as best you can, but don't worry. You can eat meals that are not balanced when you find yourself in that situation. Just know that you can be back in balance as quickly as your next meal.

Here are a few ideas to keep your diet balanced when you are designing your own meals:

Carbohydrates

- Have only one starch per meal.
- Use primarily fruits and vegetables as your main carbohydrate sources.

Protein

- Have a little protein every time you eat.
- Use high-quality, easy-to-digest protein such as eggs, egg whites, cottage cheese, skinless chicken, and turkey.

Fat

- Have some good fat at each meal.
- Use good fat like olives, olive oil, raw nuts, avocado, and fish oils.

101

USE A NUTRITION JOURNAL

I f you've never used a nutrition journal, we recommend you begin using one for the next three to six weeks. Nutrition journals are great for a number of reasons. First, they help you plan your meals. *The Formula* provides you with more than 200 meals and recipes, but not everyone likes the same thing. Use the nutrition journal to help you plan your favorite recipes.

Second, a nutrition journal can keep you motivated. Using a journal can help you track your results. In this book and *The Formula* we provide you with nutrition journals that use a star system. Record what you ate for the day (record as little or as much as you want, whatever works best for you) and give yourself a star. Try to get as many stars as possible, as often as possible. This is a simple technique to help keep you motivated and moving forward. It's like reporting in to your own personal nutrition coach. And finally, a nutrition journal will provide you with a permanent record of what you did. By reviewing your journal, you will have a record of what worked best for you.

We've been using a nutrition journal since 1984. We began using a journal when we were in mixed-pairs bodybuilding competitions. Our journals kept us motivated and opened our eyes to the combination of food and exercise that worked best for us.

It has been said that failing to plan is planning to fail. Nutrition journals are the ultimate planning tool when it comes to diet and nutrition programs. They should be enjoyable and easy to use. Use a nutrition journal to keep you motivated, to monitor your results, and to program yourself for a lifetime of better health and fitness.

Part II

THE FORMULA 101
NUTRITION JOURNAL

THE FORMULA

ACTION PLAN

Write down the time of day and the action you want to accomplish in the spaces provided. Use your action plan as a guide to help you accomplish all of your goals for the day.

TIME	GENE'S ACTION PLAN	DATE: 12-01-01
6:00 AM	wake up	
	8 oz. water	
	coffee	
7:00	breakfast	
	8 oz. water	
8:00	work	
	8 oz. water	
10:00	water break 8 oz.	
11:30	lunch	
	8 oz water	
3:30	snack	
	8 oz. water	
4:30	exercise 3-5 days a week	
	30 minutes	aerobic exercises
	20 minutes	anaerobic exercises
	20 minutes	stretching exercises
6:30	dinner	
	8 oz. water	
11:00	bed	
	8 oz. water	

SAMPLE

THE FORMULA

Write down the time of day and the action you want to accomplish in the spaces provided. Use your action plan as a guide to help you accomplish all of your goals for the day.

TIME	ACTION PLAN	DATE:

THE FORMULA

DAILY NUTRITION JOURNAL

In the spaces provided, record the date and number of the day that you have been following the Formula. Write a brief description of what you ate for the day. Using your Foumula Action Plan as your guide, give yourself a star from 1–10, 10 being your best effort and 1 being your worst. Jot down any thoughts or feelings that you have for the day.

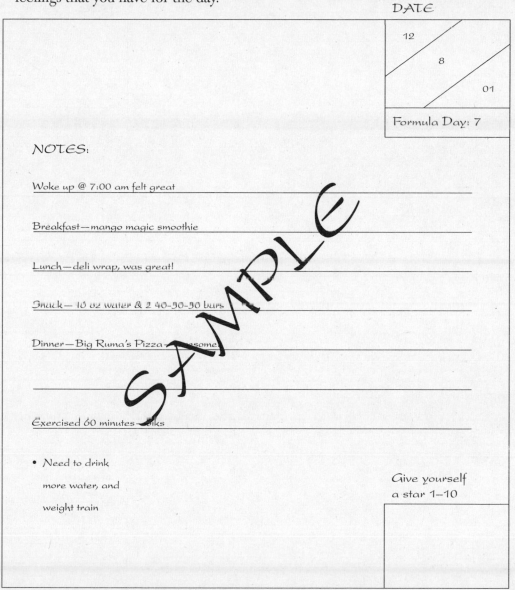

DATE

12   8   01

Formula Day: 7

NOTES:

Woke up @ 7:00 am felt great

Breakfast—mango magic smoothie

Lunch—deli wrap, was great!

Snack—16 oz water & 2 40-30-30 bars

Dinner—Big Ruma's Pizza—awsome!

Exercised 60 minutes—biks

• Need to drink
  more water, and
  weight train

Give yourself
a star 1–10

THE FORMULA

DAILY NUTRITION JOURNAL

In the spaces provided, record the date and number of the day that you have been following the Formula. Write a brief description of what you ate for the day. Using your Foumula Action Plan as your guide, give yourself a star from 1–10, 10 being your best effort and 1 being your worst. Jot down any thoughts or feelings that you have for the day.

DATE

Formula Day:

NOTES:

_____

_____

_____

_____

_____

_____

Give yourself
a star 1–10

THE FORMULA

In the spaces provided, record the date and number of the day that you have been following the Formula. Write a brief description of what you ate for the day. Using your Foumula Action Plan as your guide, give yourself a star from 1–10, 10 being your best effort and 1 being your worst. Jot down any thoughts or feelings that you have for the day.

DATE

Formula Day:

NOTES:

Give yourself
a star 1–10

THE FORMULA

In the spaces provided, record the date and number of the day that you have been following the Formula. Write a brief description of what you ate for the day. Using your Foumula Action Plan as your guide, give yourself a star from 1–10, 10 being your best effort and 1 being your worst. Jot down any thoughts or feelings that you have for the day.

DATE

Formula Day:

NOTES:

_____

_____

_____

_____

_____

_____

Give yourself
a star 1–10

THE FORMULA

In the spaces provided, record the date and number of the day that you have been following the Formula. Write a brief description of what you ate for the day. Using your Foumula Action Plan as your guide, give yourself a star from 1–10, 10 being your best effort and 1 being your worst. Jot down any thoughts or feelings that you have for the day.

DATE

Formula Day:

NOTES:

_____

_____

_____

_____

_____

_____

Give yourself
a star 1–10

THE FORMULA

In the spaces provided, record the date and number of the day that you have been following the Formula. Write a brief description of what you ate for the day. Using your Foumula Action Plan as your guide, give yourself a star from 1–10, 10 being your best effort and 1 being your worst. Jot down any thoughts or feelings that you have for the day.

DATE

Formula Day:

NOTES:

_____

_____

_____

_____

_____

_____

Give yourself
a star 1–10

THE FORMULA

DAILY NUTRITION JOURNAL

In the spaces provided, record the date and number of the day that you have been following the Formula. Write a brief description of what you ate for the day. Using your Foumula Action Plan as your guide, give yourself a star from 1–10, 10 being your best effort and 1 being your worst. Jot down any thoughts or feelings that you have for the day.

DATE

Formula Day:

NOTES:

_____

_____

_____

_____

_____

_____

Give yourself a star 1–10

THE FORMULA

In the spaces provided, record the date and number of the day that you have been following the Formula. Write a brief description of what you ate for the day. Using your Foumula Action Plan as your guide, give yourself a star from 1–10, 10 being your best effort and 1 being your worst. Jot down any thoughts or feelings that you have for the day.

DATE

Formula Day:

NOTES:

_____

_____

_____

_____

_____

_____

Give yourself
a star 1–10

THE FORMULA

DAILY NUTRITION JOURNAL

In the spaces provided, record the date and number of the day that you have been following the Formula. Write a brief description of what you ate for the day. Using your Foumula Action Plan as your guide, give yourself a star from 1–10, 10 being your best effort and 1 being your worst. Jot down any thoughts or feelings that you have for the day.

DATE

Formula Day:

NOTES:

_____

_____

_____

_____

_____

_____

Give yourself
a star 1–10

THE FORMULA

In the spaces provided, record the date and number of the day that you have been following the Formula. Write a brief description of what you ate for the day. Using your Foumula Action Plan as your guide, give yourself a star from 1–10, 10 being your best effort and 1 being your worst. Jot down any thoughts or feelings that you have for the day.

DATE

Formula Day:

NOTES:

_____

_____

_____

_____

_____

_____

Give yourself
a star 1–10

THE FORMULA

DAILY NUTRITION JOURNAL

In the spaces provided, record the date and number of the day that you have been following the Formula. Write a brief description of what you ate for the day. Using your Foumula Action Plan as your guide, give yourself a star from 1–10, 10 being your best effort and 1 being your worst. Jot down any thoughts or feelings that you have for the day.

DATE

Formula Day:

NOTES:

_____

_____

_____

_____

_____

_____

Give yourself
a star 1–10

THE FORMULA

DAILY NUTRITION JOURNAL

In the spaces provided, record the date and number of the day that you have been following the Formula. Write a brief description of what you ate for the day. Using your Foumula Action Plan as your guide, give yourself a star from 1–10, 10 being your best effort and 1 being your worst. Jot down any thoughts or feelings that you have for the day.

DATE

Formula Day:

NOTES:

Give yourself
a star 1–10

THE FORMULA

DAILY NUTRITION JOURNAL

In the spaces provided, record the date and number of the day that you have been following the Formula. Write a brief description of what you ate for the day. Using your Foumula Action Plan as your guide, give yourself a star from 1–10, 10 being your best effort and 1 being your worst. Jot down any thoughts or feelings that you have for the day.

DATE

Formula Day:

NOTES:

_____

_____

_____

_____

_____

_____

Give yourself
a star 1–10

THE FORMULA

DAILY NUTRITION JOURNAL

In the spaces provided, record the date and number of the day that you have been following the Formula. Write a brief description of what you ate for the day. Using your Foumula Action Plan as your guide, give yourself a star from 1–10, 10 being your best effort and 1 being your worst. Jot down any thoughts or feelings that you have for the day.

DATE

Formula Day:

NOTES:

_____

_____

_____

_____

_____

_____

Give yourself
a star 1–10

THE FORMULA

DAILY NUTRITION JOURNAL

In the spaces provided, record the date and number of the day that you have been following the Formula. Write a brief description of what you ate for the day. Using your Foumula Action Plan as your guide, give yourself a star from 1–10, 10 being your best effort and 1 being your worst. Jot down any thoughts or feelings that you have for the day.

DATE

Formula Day:

NOTES:

Give yourself
a star 1–10

THE FORMULA

DAILY NUTRITION JOURNAL

In the spaces provided, record the date and number of the day that you have been following the Formula. Write a brief description of what you ate for the day. Using your Foumula Action Plan as your guide, give yourself a star from 1–10, 10 being your best effort and 1 being your worst. Jot down any thoughts or feelings that you have for the day.

DATE

Formula Day:

NOTES:

_____

_____

_____

_____

_____

_____

Give yourself
a star 1–10

THE FORMULA

In the spaces provided, record the date and number of the day that you have been following the Formula. Write a brief description of what you ate for the day. Using your Foumula Action Plan as your guide, give yourself a star from 1–10, 10 being your best effort and 1 being your worst. Jot down any thoughts or feelings that you have for the day.

DATE

Formula Day:

NOTES:

_____

_____

_____

_____

_____

_____

Give yourself
a star 1–10

THE FORMULA

DAILY NUTRITION JOURNAL

In the spaces provided, record the date and number of the day that you have been following the Formula. Write a brief description of what you ate for the day. Using your Foumula Action Plan as your guide, give yourself a star from 1–10, 10 being your best effort and 1 being your worst. Jot down any thoughts or feelings that you have for the day.

DATE

Formula Day:

NOTES:

_____

_____

_____

_____

_____

_____

Give yourself
a star 1–10

THE FORMULA

DAILY NUTRITION JOURNAL

In the spaces provided, record the date and number of the day that you have been following the Formula. Write a brief description of what you ate for the day. Using your Foumula Action Plan as your guide, give yourself a star from 1–10, 10 being your best effort and 1 being your worst. Jot down any thoughts or feelings that you have for the day.

DATE

Formula Day:

NOTES:

_____

_____

_____

_____

_____

_____

Give yourself
a star 1–10

THE FORMULA

DAILY NUTRITION JOURNAL

In the spaces provided, record the date and number of the day that you have been following the Formula. Write a brief description of what you ate for the day. Using your Foumula Action Plan as your guide, give yourself a star from 1–10, 10 being your best effort and 1 being your worst. Jot down any thoughts or feelings that you have for the day.

DATE

Formula Day:

NOTES:

_____

_____

_____

_____

_____

_____

Give yourself
a star 1–10

THE FORMULA

DAILY NUTRITION JOURNAL

In the spaces provided, record the date and number of the day that you have been following the Formula. Write a brief description of what you ate for the day. Using your Foumula Action Plan as your guide, give yourself a star from 1–10, 10 being your best effort and 1 being your worst. Jot down any thoughts or feelings that you have for the day.

DATE

Formula Day:

NOTES:

Give yourself
a star 1–10

THE FORMULA
DAILY NUTRITION JOURNAL

In the spaces provided, record the date and number of the day that you have been following the Formula. Write a brief description of what you ate for the day. Using your Foumula Action Plan as your guide, give yourself a star from 1–10, 10 being your best effort and 1 being your worst. Jot down any thoughts or feelings that you have for the day.

DATE

Formula Day:

NOTES:

Give yourself
a star 1–10

THE FORMULA

DAILY NUTRITION JOURNAL

In the spaces provided, record the date and number of the day that you have been following the Formula. Write a brief description of what you ate for the day. Using your Foumula Action Plan as your guide, give yourself a star from 1–10, 10 being your best effort and 1 being your worst. Jot down any thoughts or feelings that you have for the day.

DATE

Formula Day:

NOTES:

_____

_____

_____

_____

_____

_____

Give yourself
a star 1–10

THE FORMULA

DAILY NUTRITION JOURNAL

In the spaces provided, record the date and number of the day that you have been following the Formula. Write a brief description of what you ate for the day. Using your Foumula Action Plan as your guide, give yourself a star from 1–10, 10 being your best effort and 1 being your worst. Jot down any thoughts or feelings that you have for the day.

DATE

Formula Day:

NOTES:

Give yourself
a star 1–10

THE FORMULA

DAILY NUTRITION JOURNAL

In the spaces provided, record the date and number of the day that you have been following the Formula. Write a brief description of what you ate for the day. Using your Foumula Action Plan as your guide, give yourself a star from 1–10, 10 being your best effort and 1 being your worst. Jot down any thoughts or feelings that you have for the day.

DATE

Formula Day:

NOTES:

_____

_____

_____

_____

_____

_____

Give yourself
a star 1–10

THE FORMULA

In the spaces provided, record the date and number of the day that you have been following the Formula. Write a brief description of what you ate for the day. Using your Foumula Action Plan as your guide, give yourself a star from 1–10, 10 being your best effort and 1 being your worst. Jot down any thoughts or feelings that you have for the day.

DATE

Formula Day:

NOTES:

_____

_____

_____

_____

_____

_____

Give yourself
a star 1–10

THE FORMULA

DAILY NUTRITION JOURNAL

In the spaces provided, record the date and number of the day that you have been following the Formula. Write a brief description of what you ate for the day. Using your Foumula Action Plan as your guide, give yourself a star from 1–10, 10 being your best effort and 1 being your worst. Jot down any thoughts or feelings that you have for the day.

DATE

Formula Day:

NOTES:

_____

_____

_____

_____

_____

_____

Give yourself
a star 1–10

THE FORMULA

DAILY NUTRITION JOURNAL

In the spaces provided, record the date and number of the day that you have been following the Formula. Write a brief description of what you ate for the day. Using your Foumula Action Plan as your guide, give yourself a star from 1–10, 10 being your best effort and 1 being your worst. Jot down any thoughts or feelings that you have for the day.

DATE

Formula Day:

NOTES:

_____

_____

_____

_____

_____

_____

Give yourself
a star 1–10

THE FORMULA

DAILY NUTRITION JOURNAL

In the spaces provided, record the date and number of the day that you have been following the Formula. Write a brief description of what you ate for the day. Using your Foumula Action Plan as your guide, give yourself a star from 1–10, 10 being your best effort and 1 being your worst. Jot down any thoughts or feelings that you have for the day.

DATE

Formula Day:

NOTES:

_____

_____

_____

_____

_____

_____

Give yourself
a star 1–10

THE FORMULA

DAILY NUTRITION JOURNAL

In the spaces provided, record the date and number of the day that you have
been following the Formula. Write a brief description of what you ate for the
day. Using your Foumula Action Plan as your guide, give yourself a star from
1–10, 10 being your best effort and 1 being your worst. Jot down any thoughts or
feelings that you have for the day.

DATE

Formula Day:

NOTES:

Give yourself
a star 1–10

THE FORMULA

DAILY NUTRITION JOURNAL

In the spaces provided, record the date and number of the day that you have
been following the Formula. Write a brief description of what you ate for the
day. Using your Foumula Action Plan as your guide, give yourself a star from
1–10, 10 being your best effort and 1 being your worst. Jot down any thoughts or
feelings that you have for the day.

DATE

Formula Day:

NOTES:

Give yourself
a star 1–10

THE FORMULA

DAILY NUTRITION JOURNAL

In the spaces provided, record the date and number of the day that you have
been following the Formula. Write a brief description of what you ate for the
day. Using your Foumula Action Plan as your guide, give yourself a star from
1–10, 10 being your best effort and 1 being your worst. Jot down any thoughts or
feelings that you have for the day.

DATE

Formula Day:

NOTES:

_____

_____

_____

_____

_____

_____

Give yourself
a star 1–10

THE FORMULA

MONTHLY STAR-TRACKER

In the spaces provided, record the date and number of the day that you have been following The Formula. Using your Daily Nutrition Journal as your guide, give yourself a star from 1–10, 10 being your best effort and 1 being your worst effort. Jot down any thoughts or feelings you have for the day.

MONTH: DECEMBER   YEAR: 2001

Monday	Tuesday	Wednesday	Thursday	Friday	Saturday	Sunday
					1	2
*Lost 5 lbs of fat this month and gained 8 lbs of muscle					OK Day	OK Day
___ stars	___ stars	___ stars	___ stars	___ stars	8 stars	7 stars
3	4	5	6	7	8	9
Bad Day	Great Day Felt Great	Awesome Day!	Great Day	Great Day	Great Day	Awesome Day
6 stars	9 stars	9 stars	9 stars	9 stars	9 stars	9 stars
10	11	12	13	14	15	16
Good Da more water	Good Day	Good Day	Good Day	Good Day	Good Day	Good Day
8 stars	8 stars	8 stars	8 stars	8 stars	8 stars	8 stars
17	18	19	20	21	22	23
OK Day	OK Day	Awesome Day	Good Day	Great Day	Great Day	Great Day
7 stars	7 stars	9 stars	8 stars	9 stars	9 stars	9 stars
24	25	26	27	28	29	30
OK Da	Great Day!	OK Day	Good Day	Awesome! Day	Great Day	Great Day
7 stars	9 stars	7 stars	8 stars	9 stars	9 stars	9 stars

THE FORMULA

In the spaces provided, record the date and number of the day that you have been following The Formula. Using your Daily Nutrition Journal as your guide, give yourself a star from 1–10, 10 being your best effort and 1 being your worst effort. Jot down any thoughts or feelings you have for the day.

MONTH: YEAR:

Monday	Tuesday	Wednesday	Thursday	Friday	Saturday	Sunday
___ stars	___ stars	___ stars	___ stars	___ stars	___ stars	___ stars
___ stars	___ stars	___ stars	___ stars	___ stars	___ stars	___ stars
___ stars	___ stars	___ stars	___ stars	___ stars	___ stars	___ stars
___ stars	___ stars	___ stars	___ stars	___ stars	___ stars	___ stars
___ stars	___ stars	___ stars	___ stars	___ stars	___ stars	___ stars

APPENDIXES

APPENDIX A:
THE FORMULA
MEAL PLAN SELECTION CHART

W O M E N

Activity Level	Low–Moderate	Medium–High
Hours of exercise per week	Exercise 0–4 hours per week	Exercise 5–10 hours per week
Current body weight	*Use Meal Planner*	*Use Meal Planner*
Under 140	A	B
141–180	B	C
181–200+	C	D

M E N

Activity Level	Low–Moderate	Medium–High
Hours of exercise per week	Exercise 0–4 hours per week	Exercise 5–10 hours per week
Current body weight	*Use Meal Planner*	*Use Meal Planner*
Under 140	B	C
141–180	C	D
181–250+	C	D

Your Personalized Meal Plan is _____

THE FORMULA

MEAL PLAN SELECTION CHART FOR ELITE ATHLETES

FEMALE ELITE ATHLETES

Current Body Weight	Train 10 or more hours per week
Under 140	C
141–180	D
180+	E

MALE ELITE ATHLETES

Current Body Weight	Train 10 or more hours per week
Under 140	C
141–180	D
180+	E

Your Personalized Meal Plan is _____

APPENDIX B:
MEAL PLANNER MACRONUTRIENT CHART

Listed below are the total grams of carbohydrate, protein, fat and calories listed for each meal plan. The meal plans have been tailored for individual requirements based on gender, weight, and activity levels. To determine which meal plan is right for you, refer to *The Formula Meal Plan Selection Chart*. Each meal and snack contains the 40-30-30 ratio, which provides 40% of its *total calories* from carbohydrates, 30% from protein, and 30% from fat.

Personal Meal Plan	A	B	C	D	E
BREAKFAST					
Carbohydrate grams	20	20	33	47	53
Protein grams	15	15	25	35	40
Fat grams	6	6	11	13	18
Calories	194	194	331	445	534
LUNCH					
Carbohydrate grams	27	40	40	53	66
Protein grams	20	30	30	40	50
Fat grams	9	14	14	18	22
Calories	269	406	406	534	662
SNACKS					
Carbohydrate grams	20	20	20	20	40
Protein grams	15	15	15	15	30
Fat grams	6	6	6	6	12
Calories	194	194	194	194	388
DINNER					
Carbohydrate grams	40	47	53	53	66
Protein grams	30	35	40	40	50
Fat grams	14	15	18	18	22
Calories	406	463	534	534	662

Personal Meal Plan	A	B	C	D	E
DINNER					
Carbohydrate grams	40	47	53	53	66
Protein grams	30	35	40	40	50
Fat grams	14	15	18	18	22
Calories	406	463	534	534	662
DAILY TOTALS					
Carbohydrate grams	106	126	146	173	226
Protein grams	80	95	110	130	170
Fat grams	35	42	48	57	75
Calories	1,063	1,257	1,465	1,707	2,246

APPENDIX C:
SPECIAL INGREDIENTS

Pure Whey Protein Powder

Whey protein powder is a natural protein from dairy. It is lactose- and fat-free, mixes instantly and has a great amino acid profile. A high-quality whey protein powder should be 90% pure protein and contain no added sweeteners or flavors. Pure whey protein is sometimes hard to find. The brand we use and feel is one of the best available is Pure WPI by Bioplex Nutrition. It can be found in quality health food stores. If you have trouble finding Pure WPI or a comparable protein powder in your area, you can order it from Craig Nutraceuticals (a nutritional foods mail order company) at 1-800-293-1683

Granulated Fructose

Granulated fructose is a granulated fruit sugar that is very low-glycemic. It is available in most health food stores and many grocery stores.

ABOUT THE AUTHORS

Gene and Joyce Daoust are the authors of the national bestseller *The Formula*. They are two of the original nutritionists who helped develop and test the 40-30-30 zone nutrition program. In 1992, the Daousts opened the Bio Syn Human Performance Center, a cutting-edge weight-loss and sports-nutrition facility and the world's first 40-30-30 zone nutrition clinic. The Daousts frequently appear as featured speakers and conduct programs for corporations nationwide.